NURSOPATHIC MEDICINE

A Theoretical Framework for Autonomous Nursing Practice

LAZARO GAFAS
MSN, ARNP, FNP-C, PMHNP-BC

MIAMI MENTAL HEALTH

Nursopathic Medicine
A Theoretical Framework for Autonomous Nursing Practice

Published by Miami Mental Health
Miami, Florida

First Edition, 2026

ISBN (Paperback): 979-8-9947601-0-9
ISBN (Ebook): 979-8-9947601-1-6

Cover design & typesetting by Islam Farid

Printed in the United States of America

Trademark Notices

Citation Information

To cite this book (APA 7th edition format): Gafas, L. (2026). *Nursopathic medicine: A theoretical framework for autonomous nursing practice*. Miami Mental Health.

To cite a specific chapter: Gafas, L. (2026). [Chapter title]. In *Nursopathic medicine: A theoretical framework for autonomous nursing practice* (pp. [page range]). Miami Mental Health.

Availability

Available in paperback and ebook editions through: Amazon (Paperback & Kindle), Barnes & Noble (Paperback & NOOK) and other major book retailers.
For updates or supplementary materials, visit: **miamentalhealth.com**

Contact and Permissions

For book-related inquiries, speaking engagements, media requests, or to request permission to reproduce selections from this book, contact:

Miami Mental Health
Psychiatric-Mental Health Services
Miami, Florida

Email: **info@miamentalhealth.com**
Website: **miamentalhealth.com**

When requesting permission to reproduce material, please include:
Title of the work,
Specific material to be reproduced,
Number of copies to be made,
Intended use and distribution.

Disclaimer

This book is intended for educational purposes for nurse practitioner students, practicing nurse practitioners, nursing faculty, healthcare administrators, policymakers, and other professionals interested in understanding the theoretical foundations of autonomous advanced practice nursing.

While the content is based on current evidence, professional standards, and the author's clinical and academic expertise, it should not be construed as legal advice, medical advice, or definitive guidance for individual practice situations. Healthcare regulations, scope of practice laws, and clinical standards vary by jurisdiction and evolve over time.

Readers are responsible for:

- Consulting current federal and state regulations applicable to their practice location
- Following institutional policies and procedures
- Adhering to their professional licensure and certification requirements
- Exercising independent professional judgment appropriate to their education, experience, and scope of practice
- Seeking legal counsel when regulatory or scope of practice questions arise

The author and publisher specifically disclaim any liability, loss, or risk, personal or otherwise, incurred as a consequence, directly or indirectly, of the use and application of any of the contents of this book.

Professional Practice Responsibility: Each nurse practitioner is responsible for practicing within their individual scope of practice as determined by their education, certification, state licensure, and competency. This book provides a theoretical framework and does not expand or restrict any individual practitioner's legal scope of practice.

The views and opinions expressed in this book are those of the author and do not necessarily reflect the official policy or position of any healthcare organization, regulatory body, professional association, or certifying agency.

Acknowledgment of Artificial Intelligence Assistance

This work was developed in collaboration with Claude, an artificial intelligence system created by Anthropic. The nature and extent of that collaboration is described precisely below.

All clinical expertise, nursing knowledge, theoretical frameworks, professional insights, and substantive content are the original work of the author, Lazaro Gafas, MSN, ARNP, FNP-C, PMHNP-BC. The author takes full responsibility for the accuracy, completeness, and professional integrity of all content presented.

The use of AI assistance was employed to:

- Organize the author's clinical and theoretical ideas into manuscript structure and chapter sequencing
- Draft and refine prose from the author's outlined arguments, clinical examples, and theoretical positions
- Develop practice questions and case studies based on the author's clinical scenarios and learning objectives
- Identify and correct internal inconsistencies in scope, terminology, and cross-references
- The theoretical framework, clinical expertise, professional arguments, and substantive intellectual content originate with the author. The author reviewed, revised, and takes full responsibility for all content.

Dedication

To the memory of my mother,
Osmara Borrero
(1970-2019)

Your struggle with mental illness and loss to suicide
taught me that psychiatric care demands
the highest level of expertise, compassion, and autonomy.

The nurse practitioners who care for patients like you
deserve clear professional frameworks,
autonomous authority, and recognition
for the life-saving work they do.

This book is dedicated to your memory
and to advancing the care of all who suffer
from illnesses that are too often invisible,
stigmatized, or undertreated.

Your life mattered. Your struggle mattered.
May this work honor your memory
by strengthening the profession that serves
those who walk the path you walked.

I love you and miss you.

ACKNOWLEDGMENTS

This book represents the culmination of ideas I have carried for years: ideas about what it means to practice as a nurse practitioner, how to articulate our professional identity, and how to explain autonomous practice in terms grounded in nursing itself. While the concepts are mine, their organization and expression owe much to collaboration, support, and the quiet encouragement of those who believed this work mattered.

To my wife and son: thank you for your patience, understanding, and unwavering support throughout the countless hours I spent immersed in this work. You gave me the space to think, write, and refine these ideas, and you listened with grace to more conversations about "nursopathic medicine" than anyone should reasonably endure. Your belief in this project sustained me when the path forward seemed unclear. This book exists because you made room for it in our lives.

I am deeply grateful to my best friend, Ernesto Yglesias, MSN, ARNP, FNP-C, BCBA-BC, who has been my moral support and father figure throughout this journey. His unwavering encouragement and wisdom have been invaluable, and I cannot imagine completing this work without his guidance and friendship.

I also extend my heartfelt thanks to Dr. Monica Barfield, DNP, APRN, AGACNP-BC, FNP-BC, whose practice at New Horizon Primary Care in Port St. Joe, Florida exemplifies the five domains of this framework in action. Her work in rural primary care demonstrates what autonomous nursing practice looks like when it is grounded in clinical excellence, patient-centered care, and unwavering advocacy for the communities nurse practitioners serve. Her collaborative spirit and commitment to advancing the profession have been an inspiration.

To my close friends and colleagues who offered encouragement, critical feedback, and moral support: your insights sharpened my thinking and your confidence in this work kept me moving forward. You listened to early drafts, challenged my assumptions, and reminded me why this theoretical work matters for our profession. I am grateful for your friendship and your commitment to advancing nursing practice.

Finally, I want to honor those who have worked tirelessly behind the scenes (advocates, educators, policymakers, researchers, and countless nurse practitioners) fighting for full practice authority, professional recognition, and the right of our profession to define itself on its own terms. You have challenged restrictive regulations, educated legislators, published research, mentored students, and defended the legitimacy of autonomous practice in boardrooms, legislatures, and clinical settings. Your efforts often go unrecognized, your victories hard-won and incremental.

This book is intended as a drop of water in the vast ocean of advocacy you have built. It offers a theoretical framework for something you have already proven in practice: that nurse practitioners can and do practice autonomously with competence, accountability, and integrity. May it provide our profession with one more tool (a conceptual language) to articulate what you have long demonstrated through your work.

If this book helps even one nurse practitioner explain their practice with greater clarity, supports one educator in teaching professional identity with confidence, or provides one policymaker with a nursing-centered framework for understanding autonomous practice, it will have fulfilled its purpose.

To all who contributed to this work, directly or indirectly: thank you. This is our collective effort to define our profession in our own terms.

LAZARO GAFAS, MSN, ARNP, FNP-C, PMHNP-BC
2026

PREFACE

This book addresses a conceptual gap in nursing theory: the absence of a coherent framework explaining how nurse practitioners practice medicine autonomously through advanced nursing practice. While autonomous practice has become an established feature of contemporary healthcare delivery, it remains insufficiently defined within nursing's theoretical foundations.

Nursopathic medicine is proposed as a unifying framework that explains autonomous nurse practitioner practice through five functional domains: Acute Care, Chronic Care, Preventative Care, Interdisciplinary Care, and Specialty Care. These domains rest upon a foundation of evidence-based practice and describe how nurse practitioners exercise clinical authority across diverse settings and populations.

Author's Note: How This Framework Emerged from Practice

The conceptual formation of the Nursopathic Medicine Practice Model emerged not from abstract theorizing but from systematic observation of nurse practitioner practice patterns across multiple clinical settings. I graduated from the University of Miami with my Family Nurse Practitioner certification in 2016 and completed my post-master's Psychiatric-Mental Health Nurse Practitioner certificate, also at UM, in 2022. Over those years of practice, I recognized patterns in how I and my colleagues approached clinical work—patterns that existing nursing theories didn't adequately explain.

Whether working in primary care or psychiatric practice, whether consulting with family NPs, acute care NPs, or psychiatric NPs, I observed the same functional structure underlying autonomous practice. We all navigated acute clinical presentations requiring timely assessment and intervention. We all provided longitudinal management of chronic conditions. We all engaged in preventative screening and risk reduction. We all coordinated care across interdisciplinary teams. And we all applied specialized knowledge to defined patient populations or clinical domains. These weren't arbitrary categories I invented—they were consistent domains through which autonomous NP practice actually operates, regardless of specialty.

As a primary care and family practice nurse practitioner, my clinical days naturally rotated through what would later become the five domains. I managed acute presentations—walk-in complaints, urgent symptoms requiring same-day assessment and treatment decisions. I provided chronic disease management for patients with diabetes, hypertension, and heart failure, adjusting medications and monitoring outcomes over time. I engaged in preventative care, driven partly by workplace HEDIS (Healthcare Effectiveness Data and Information Set) measures and Medicare Risk Adjustment (MRA) coding requirements—screening for colorectal cancer, ordering mammograms, performing depression screenings, ensuring age-appropriate immunizations.

Interdisciplinary care was constant. I referred patients to specialists for colonoscopies, mammograms, colposcopies, and subspecialty consultation when conditions exceeded my scope or required advanced intervention. Later, as a PMHNP, I would practice this domain in reverse—referring patients back to their primary care providers for metabolic monitoring of antipsychotic medications or coordinating with cardiologists when psychiatric medications posed cardiovascular concerns.

Specialty care manifested differently across these roles. In family practice, my population focus was lifespan primary care. In psychiatric practice, my specialty became mental health assessment, diagnosis, and psychopharmacology. The specificity of knowledge differed, but the function remained consistent: applying advanced, focused expertise to a defined patient population or clinical domain.

I tested this observation systematically. I discussed practice patterns with colleagues across specialties. I analyzed how NPs described their work in professional forums and job descriptions. I reviewed scope of practice literature and regulatory frameworks. The pattern held. Regardless of specialty—family practice, psychiatric, acute care, pediatrics, women's health—NPs described navigating the same five functional domains with different clinical content. The framework wasn't describing my idiosyncratic practice—it was revealing the shared structure underlying autonomous nurse practitioner work.

Throughout this observation period, I maintained engagement with evidence-based practice, regularly consulting UpToDate and Epocrates for current clinical guidelines. I watched those guidelines evolve in real time, and my practice evolved with them. I remember when the standard treatment for chlamydia was azithromycin 1 gram as a single dose—favored for its simplicity and presumed better compliance. That guideline remained standard from 2016 through 2021.

But I noticed something in my own patient population: many returned weeks later with the same symptoms. While reinfection was possible, the pattern suggested treatment failure rates higher than expected. I began switching to doxycycline 100 mg twice daily for seven days—at the time considered second-line treatment—and observed better clinical outcomes. My clinical judgment, informed by direct observation of treatment effectiveness, led me to deviate from the guideline before formal evidence supported that decision. In July 2021, the CDC released updated STI Treatment Guidelines officially changing the first-line recommendation to doxycycline, citing emerging azithromycin resistance and higher cure rates with doxycycline. This experience reinforced a fundamental aspect of autonomous practice: evidence-based care requires critical evaluation of outcomes, not just algorithmic compliance with guidelines.

Existing nursing theories—from Peplau's interpersonal theory to Watson's caring science to Benner's novice-to-expert framework—describe important aspects of nursing values, relationships, and expertise development. But they don't adequately explain the functional structure of autonomous advanced practice nursing. They don't clarify how nurse practitioners exercise independent diagnostic and therapeutic authority. They don't delineate the specific domains through which NP practice operates or explain how those domains differ from basic nursing practice or physician practice. This theoretical gap leaves nurse practitioners without clear language to articulate what we do when we practice autonomously—a gap that contributes to the conceptual confusion described throughout this book.

What I recognized through systematic observation of NP practice patterns was not my personal workflow but the underlying functional architecture that all autonomous NPs navigate. The five domains weren't invented categories imposed on practice—they were observed functional realities that emerged from analyzing how NPs actually work. What this book articulates is what thousands of nurse practitioners were already doing. The framework simply names it, organizes it, and explains why it works within a nursing rather than medical theoretical foundation.

Nursopathic medicine, in other words, is descriptive before it is prescriptive. It explains existing autonomous NP practice rather than dictating how practice should occur. That's why it resonates: because it describes what nurse practitioners already know from lived experience, even when we lack the theoretical language to articulate it clearly. If this framework feels familiar as you read it, it's because you're likely already practicing within these domains. This book provides the conceptual tools to explain, defend, and advance what you already do.

> *This book articulates what emerged from systematic observation of nurse practitioner practice patterns rather than what I imagined through abstract theorizing. The five domains were not invented—they were recognized as the functional structure underlying autonomous NP work across specialties and settings. What follows is an attempt to explain, organize, and defend what nurse practitioners already do when we practice autonomously, using a theoretical framework that addresses the conceptual gaps existing nursing theories have left unfilled. If this framework resonates, it is because you recognize your own practice within it.*

Important Clarification

Nursopathic medicine applies specifically to nurse practitioner practice at the advanced practice registered nurse (APRN) level. It describes a practice model centered on autonomous diagnostic and therapeutic decision-making (the core activity that distinguishes nurse practitioner practice from other APRN roles). Certified nurse midwives engage in diagnostic and therapeutic practice within their reproductive and women's health scope, and will find significant resonance with this framework within that context. Certified registered nurse anesthetists and clinical nurse specialists, however, operate under fundamentally different practice models. Anesthesia practice is organized around perioperative patient management rather than the independent diagnostic-therapeutic cycle this framework addresses. Clinical nurse specialist practice traditionally emphasizes consultation, education, and systems-level improvement rather than direct autonomous patient management. These are distinct and essential contributions to nursing. Nursopathic medicine does not diminish them; it simply describes a different practice model, one that is specific to the way nurse practitioners engage in medicine through a nursing framework. It does not describe registered nursing practice, which operates under a different scope of practice, authority structure, and model of accountability.

The purpose of this framework is not to advocate for scope expansion or regulatory change, but to provide nursing with an internally coherent explanation of advanced practice as it currently exists. By articulating how nurse practitioners reason, collaborate, and maintain accountability, this model supports clarity in education, consistency in regulation, and stability in professional identity.

This text is intended primarily for nurse practitioner students and practicing nurse practitioners, as well as educators, policymakers, and scholars interested in understanding the theoretical foundations of autonomous nursing practice. Certified nurse midwives and other APRNs whose practice encompasses diagnostic and therapeutic decision-making will find the framework applicable within their respective scopes.

A Note on Examples

Clinical examples throughout this text focus on nurse practitioner practice, which constitutes the largest APRN group and encompasses the widest variety of practice settings in which the five-domain framework applies. Certified nurse midwives will find the framework particularly applicable within reproductive and women's health contexts, where the diagnostic-therapeutic practice model this text describes is fully represented.

HOW TO USE THIS BOOK

This textbook is organized into four parts that progress from foundational concepts to practical application:

Part I: Foundations establishes the problem of autonomous practice, traces the historical development of the nurse practitioner role, and introduces nursopathic medicine as a conceptual solution.

Part II: The Nursopathic Medicine Practice Model presents the theoretical framework organizing autonomous practice into five functional domains supported by evidence-based practice.

Part III: The Five Domains of Practice provides detailed examination of each domain (Acute Care, Chronic Care, Preventative Care, Interdisciplinary Care, and Specialty Care) with applications across specialties.

Part IV: Synthesis and Implications explores the ethical foundations, regulatory implications, and future directions for autonomous nursing practice.

Each chapter includes:

- Learning objectives
- Core content with clear headings
- Illustrative examples across specialties
- Chapter summaries
- Critical thinking questions

Readers may approach this text linearly or focus on specific domains relevant to their practice setting. Educators may use individual chapters as standalone readings or integrate the complete framework into advanced practice curricula.

CONTENTS

PART I

FOUNDATIONS OF AUTONOMOUS PRACTICE

CHAPTER 1

THE PROBLEM OF AUTONOMOUS PRACTICE

LEARNING OBJECTIVES

Upon completing this chapter, students will be able to:

Define autonomous practice and distinguish it from collaborative or delegated practice models.

Explain the conceptual gap between regulatory recognition and theoretical explanation of nurse practitioner autonomous practice.

Identify at least three consequences of conceptual ambiguity in advanced nursing practice.

Analyze how the absence of nursing-centered frameworks affects professional identity, education, and policy.

Describe the shared clinical space where nurse practitioners and physicians exercise overlapping authority.

Evaluate why historical and legal justifications alone are insufficient for explaining contemporary NP practice.

Articulate the central problem this book addresses: how autonomous authority is understood rather than whether it exists.

CRITICAL THINKING QUESTIONS

Analysis: How does the conceptual gap between what nurse practitioners do and how their practice is theoretically explained create vulnerabilities in policy debates? Provide specific examples.

Application: Consider a nurse practitioner working in a state with full practice authority. Even with legal autonomy, how might the absence of theoretical clarity affect their professional identity or interprofessional relationships?

Evaluation: The chapter states that autonomous practice may be "interpreted variably (as collaboration, delegation, substitution, or exception) rather than as a legitimate and stable mode of advanced nursing practice." Which of these interpretations is most problematic, and why?

Synthesis: Imagine you're explaining to a nursing student why nurse practitioners need a theoretical framework beyond just having legal authority to practice. What would you say?

Comparison: How does the problem described in this chapter differ from questions about NP competence or clinical outcomes? Why is this distinction important?

Reflection: Have you observed or experienced situations where ambiguity about NP autonomous practice created confusion or conflict? How might theoretical clarity have helped?

Debate: Some might argue, "If NPs are legally allowed to practice autonomously and patient outcomes are good, why does theoretical explanation matter?" How would you respond?

1. INTRODUCTION

Autonomous practice by nurse practitioners is an established feature of contemporary healthcare delivery, yet it remains insufficiently defined within nursing theory. In primary care and specialty settings alike, nurse practitioners independently evaluate patients, establish diagnoses, initiate treatment plans, prescribe medications, and assume responsibility for clinical outcomes (Institute of Medicine, 2011; Fairman et al., 2011). These activities are recognized through licensure, regulation, and institutional policy. However, the conceptual framework explaining how such authority functions within nursing has not evolved at the same pace as practice itself.

This book focuses on nurse practitioner practice at the advanced practice registered nurse (APRN) level. Nursopathic medicine applies specifically to nurse practitioner practice. The APRN role in which autonomous diagnostic and therapeutic decision-making is the defining feature of clinical activity. It does not describe registered nursing practice, which operates under a different scope of practice, authority structure, and model of accountability. The precise boundaries of this framework, and why it addresses nurse practitioner practice specifically rather than all APRN roles, are examined in detail below.

NP AUTONOMOUS PRACTICE EXISTS

- 50 states license NPs
- 30+ states grant full authority
- Decades of evidence supporting safety/effectiveness

↓

BUT: CONCEPTUAL GAP

Nursing lacks theoretical framework explaining HOW autonomous practice functions as nursing

↓

CONSEQUENCES

- Professional identity confusion
- Regulatory vulnerability
- Educational inconsistency
- Interprofessional misunderstanding

↓

SOLUTION: NURSOPATHIC MEDICINE

Five functional domains explaining autonomous practice through nursing framework

Figure 1.1. The Problem of Autonomous Practice and Its Solution

2. THE CONCEPTUAL GAP IN NURSING THEORY

Historically, nursing theory has emphasized relational care, collaboration, and role differentiation. These emphases remain central to nursing identity, yet they do not fully account for the scope and depth of decision-making authority exercised by nurse practitioners in autonomous practice environments. As a result, autonomous practice is frequently described in legal or operational terms rather than as a coherent professional model grounded in nursing epistemology.

This gap has placed nurse practitioner practice in a conceptual intermediary space. From a regulatory perspective, autonomy is defined by scope and licensure. From a clinical perspective, autonomy is expressed through independent judgment and accountability. From a theoretical perspective, however, the integration of medical diagnosis and treatment within nursing practice remains under-articulated. The absence of a unifying explanation has allowed autonomous practice to be interpreted variably (as collaboration, delegation, substitution, or exception) rather than as a legitimate and stable mode of advanced nursing practice.

3. CONSEQUENCES OF CONCEPTUAL AMBIGUITY

The consequences of this conceptual ambiguity extend beyond academic discourse. When autonomous practice lacks theoretical clarity, it becomes vulnerable to misinterpretation in policy debates, inconsistency in education, and confusion in interprofessional relationships. These challenges do not arise from deficiencies in nurse practitioner capability or outcomes, but from the absence of a nursing-centered framework that explains how medical decision-making functions within advanced nursing practice.

This ambiguity is particularly evident within contemporary clinical environments where professional roles intersect. The expansion of autonomous practice has created a shared clinical space in which nurse practitioners and physicians exercise overlapping diagnostic and therapeutic authority. In many practice settings, nurse practitioners independently evaluate patients, initiate treatment, and manage outcomes alongside allopathic and osteopathic providers. While this shared space reflects the realities of modern healthcare delivery, it also exposes unresolved conceptual tensions regarding professional authority.

4. THE CHALLENGE OF SHARED CLINICAL SPACE

In the absence of a clear nursing-centered framework for autonomous practice, overlapping scopes of clinical activity may be interpreted through historical models of medical hierarchy rather than through current regulatory and educational realities. These models were developed in different eras of professional organization and do not fully account for the evolution of advanced nursing practice. As a result, autonomous nursing practice may be viewed inconsistently across institutions and disciplines, despite clear legal recognition.

This structural ambiguity can generate professional friction that is systemic rather than interpersonal. When authority is exercised without a shared conceptual understanding, nurse practitioners may experience uncertainty regarding professional identity and legitimacy, even while bearing full responsibility for clinical decisions and patient outcomes. Such internalized uncertainty reflects a mismatch between practice authority and theoretical explanation rather than a lack of competence or preparation.

By framing autonomous practice primarily in legal or operational terms, rather than within nursing theory, the profession has left this shared clinical space conceptually underdeveloped. Clarifying how nurse practitioners practice medicine through a nursing framework is therefore essential not only for regulatory coherence, but also for professional stability within interdisciplinary environments.

5. IMPOSTER SYNDROME AND PROFESSIONAL IDENTITY

The internalized uncertainty described above manifests clinically as imposter syndrome, the persistent feeling that one's professional authority is not legitimate despite objective evidence of competence. Imposter syndrome is widely documented among nurse practitioners across specialties and experience levels, and while it is often framed as an individual psychological challenge, it reflects a deeper structural problem.

When nurse practitioners diagnose illness, prescribe medications, and manage complex patients independently, they engage in activities that have historically been associated with physicians. If nursing theory has not provided a clear explanation for how these activities function within nursing, nurse practitioners are left without a professional framework to anchor their identity. The result is a cognitive dissonance: they practice autonomously, yet lack the theoretical language to explain that their practice is nursing rather than borrowed medicine.

This dissonance does not arise from inadequate preparation or insufficient clinical skill. It arises from the conceptual gap this chapter has identified. Nurse practitioners are granted authority through licensure and regulation, educated through rigorous graduate programs, and held accountable for clinical outcomes, yet nursing has not articulated a unified theoretical explanation for how autonomous diagnostic and therapeutic practice fits within nursing epistemology. The absence of this explanation leaves nurse practitioners vulnerable to doubt, not because their practice is illegitimate, but because their profession has not yet given them the conceptual tools to understand and articulate that legitimacy.

Imposter syndrome, in this context, is not personal failure. It is a predictable response to structural ambiguity. When a profession gives its practitioners authority without theoretical grounding for that authority, practitioners internalize the gap as inadequacy. They may question whether they are "really" practicing nursing, whether their decisions are as valid as those of physicians, whether their role is legitimate or merely tolerated. These are not questions of competence, they are questions of identity, and they persist because nursing theory has not resolved them.

Nursopathic medicine addresses this by providing a nursing-centered framework that explains autonomous practice as an extension of nursing rather than an adoption of medicine. It affirms that nurse practitioners practice medicine through nursing (grounded in nursing education, nursing ethics, and nursing ways of knowing) and that this practice is coherent, defensible, and theoretically sound. By offering language and structure for what nurse practitioners already do, the framework reduces the cognitive dissonance that fuels imposter syndrome. It does not eliminate the challenges of professional development or the natural uncertainties of clinical practice, but it removes the foundational question: Is what I'm doing actually nursing?

The answer this framework provides is unequivocal: Yes. Autonomous diagnostic and therapeutic practice, when conducted within scope by nurse practitioners educated and certified for that role, is nursing. It is nursing practiced at an advanced level, integrating biomedical knowledge with nursing judgment, but it remains nursing. This clarity is not merely semantic. For many nurse practitioners, it is psychologically essential.

The structural resolution the framework provides, however, is only part of the answer. Chapter 5 addresses the developmental dimension: how imposter syndrome takes hold during the RN-to-NP transition when formation is inadequate, and how preceptorship, mentorship, and the acceptance of clinical limits build the internal grounding that allows a clinician to practice with confidence rather than doubt.

6. DEFINING THE PROBLEM

The central problem of autonomous practice, then, is not whether nurse practitioners are capable of independent clinical authority, but how that authority is understood. Without a clear theoretical account, autonomy remains defined externally (by statutes, institutional policies, or comparisons to other professions) rather than internally by nursing itself. This leaves advanced practice vulnerable to mischaracterization and dependent on frameworks that were not designed to explain nursing-based medical decision-making.

Throughout this book, the term "medicine" refers to the practice domain of diagnosing, treating, and managing disease through biomedical knowledge. Not to the exclusive practice of physicians. Nursopathic medicine describes how nurse practitioners engage in medical practice through a nursing framework, grounded in nursing education, ethics, and professional identity. This distinction is elaborated in Chapter 3.

7. WHY NURSE PRACTITIONER PRACTICE SPECIFICALLY

A natural question arises at this point: if nursopathic medicine is a nursing framework, why does it apply to nurse practitioner practice specifically rather than to all advanced practice registered nurse (APRN) roles? The answer lies in what distinguishes the nurse practitioner role from other APRNs. Not in importance or clinical rigor, but in the structure of practice itself.

The APRN designation encompasses four roles: nurse practitioners, clinical nurse specialists, certified registered nurse anesthetists, and certified nurse midwives. These roles share graduate-level preparation, national certification, and advanced clinical competence. What they do not all share is the same practice model. Nursopathic medicine is built around a specific practice model. One in which the clinician independently diagnoses, prescribes, treats, and longitudinally manages patients across the full cycle of care. This is the diagnostic-therapeutic practice model. It is the practice model that the five domains of this framework, acute care, chronic care, preventative care, interdisciplinary care, and specialty care, were designed to describe.

Nurse practitioner practice is defined by this model. In primary care and specialty settings alike, nurse practitioners independently evaluate patients, establish diagnoses, initiate and adjust treatment plans, prescribe medications, and assume accountability for clinical outcomes. This is the practice activity that nursopathic medicine describes and that the conceptual gap identified in this chapter fails to explain.

Certified nurse midwives engage in diagnostic and therapeutic practice within their reproductive and women's health scope, and this framework applies meaningfully within that context. The five domains are recognizable in midwifery practice as it functions in contemporary clinical settings.

Certified registered nurse anesthetists, by contrast, practice under a fundamentally different model. Anesthesia practice is organized around perioperative patient management. The assessment, induction, maintenance, and emergence from anesthesia, and the management of patients in the perioperative period. This is essential, high-acuity clinical work. But it does not center on the independent diagnostic-therapeutic cycle that nursopathic medicine describes. A CRNA does not typically establish a diagnosis, develop a longitudinal treatment plan, and manage a patient across the arc of a chronic condition. The practice model is different, and therefore the conceptual framework is different.

Clinical nurse specialists practice under a different model as well. The CNS role has historically emphasized indirect care (consultation, education, research utilization, and systems-level quality improvement) rather than direct autonomous patient management. While some CNS practice has evolved toward more direct patient care in certain settings, the traditional and still-predominant CNS practice model does not map onto the five-domain framework built around independent diagnostic and therapeutic authority.

This is not a hierarchy. It is a distinction. Nursopathic medicine does not describe a superior form of nursing practice (it describes a specific one. The boundary of the framework is drawn at the diagnostic-therapeutic practice model, not at the credential. Any APRN whose practice is organized around independent diagnosis, treatment, and longitudinal management is engaging in the practice this framework addresses. Nurse practitioners do so as a matter of role definition. The framework's specificity to that practice model is what gives it conceptual precision) and what allows it to answer the question this book sets out to address: how does medicine function within nursing?

8. PURPOSE OF THIS BOOK

The purpose of this book is to address this problem by articulating nursopathic medicine as a coherent model of autonomous practice. By recognizing the practice of medicine as an inherent component of advanced nursing practice, this framework provides a nursing-centered explanation for diagnosis, treatment, and longitudinal management within scope. The chapters that follow examine how this model emerged, how it functions, and why it is necessary to sustain clarity, accountability, and professional identity in contemporary healthcare.

Clinical Reflection: Navigating Shared Clinical Space as a New Graduate

I remember my first nurse practitioner job right out of school. I started working for a small private practice doing family medicine, where I was given only two weeks of training by the physician assistant who had been working there before being released to see patients on my own. It was a daunting moment—learning to practice independently without substantial guidance. Despite some early missteps, I learned quickly and valued the autonomy of working independently. Because I was functioning in a largely independent capacity, I didn't initially experience the conceptual gap I would later encounter while working as an assistant to a specialist physician.

What I did encounter, however, was a stark example of conflict within shared clinical space—both with the PA and the practice's medical director. The issue centered on a 60-year-old patient who I suspected had developed Type 1.5 diabetes, also known as Latent Autoimmune Diabetes in Adults (LADA). After performing a urinalysis showing ketosis, ordering C-peptide levels, and reviewing her hemoglobin A1C, I diagnosed LADA and initiated treatment with Lantus (long-acting insulin) while referring her to an endocrinologist.

The medical director expressed strong clinical concerns about my treatment decision. He believed that metformin was more appropriate than insulin for a patient of her age, citing standard Type 2 diabetes management approaches. His concern was genuine—he wanted to ensure patient safety and avoid potential complications from insulin therapy in what he assessed as a Type 2 presentation. The office manager supported this clinical position, recommending we follow the conventional Type 2 protocol despite the laboratory findings I believed suggested LADA.

This experience revealed something deeper than a clinical disagreement. Both the medical director and I held legitimate diagnostic and therapeutic authority over this patient. The challenge was not whose clinical judgment was superior—the endocrinologist's subsequent confirmation of LADA through autoimmune antibody testing validated my diagnostic reasoning, but that wasn't the central issue. The challenge was the absence of a framework for understanding how my nursing-based clinical assessment could operate as autonomous professional judgment rather than requiring physician approval or revision.

This wasn't about one physician being dismissive or one new graduate being overconfident. It was about a conceptual gap that left both of us uncertain about how independent clinical reasoning operates in shared clinical space. Without clarity about the boundaries and legitimacy of nurse practitioner autonomous judgment, disagreements default to hierarchical resolution: the physician's perspective supersedes the nurse practitioner's, not necessarily because of superior reasoning, but because institutional structures assume physician authority in the absence of clear alternatives.

The disagreement led to my departure from the practice. What this experience taught me was not that physicians resist nurse practitioner autonomy out of malice, but that healthcare institutions lack conceptual frameworks for understanding how autonomous clinical judgment operates when multiple professionals hold legitimate authority over the same clinical decisions. The framework for nursopathic medicine that this book articulates emerged partly from this early experience—the recognition that NP authority needs theoretical explanation, not just regulatory permission.

This experience exemplifies the "shared clinical space" concept described in this chapter. The medical director and I both held diagnostic and therapeutic authority over this patient, yet the framework for understanding how my nursing-based clinical judgment operated alongside his medical perspective was absent. The result was not collaborative refinement of clinical reasoning, but hierarchical resolution based on institutional default assumptions. Both of us were operating in good faith within a system that lacked conceptual clarity about professional boundaries.

CHAPTER SUMMARY

Autonomous nurse practitioner practice exists in a conceptual gap between regulatory recognition and theoretical explanation. This gap creates ambiguity in professional identity, education, and interprofessional relationships. The problem is not clinical competence, but the absence of a nursing-centered framework that explains how medical decision-making operates within advanced nursing practice. Nursopathic medicine is proposed as a solution to this conceptual problem.

CHAPTER 1
PRACTICE QUESTIONS

MULTIPLE CHOICE QUESTIONS

1. **The "conceptual gap" in nursing theory regarding autonomous NP practice refers to:**
   A. The difference between what NPs want to do and what regulations allow
   B. The absence of theoretical explanation for how NPs practice medicine through nursing
   C. The gap between physician and NP salaries
   D. The difference between entry-level and experienced NP competence

2. **According to Chapter 1, autonomous practice is best understood as:**
   A. Complete independence from all other healthcare professionals
   B. The ability to practice without legal restrictions
   C. Alignment of authority, responsibility, and accountability
   D. A privilege granted by physicians

3. **The chapter argues that historical justifications for NP practice (access, collaboration, delegation) are insufficient because they:**
   A. Are factually inaccurate
   B. Frame autonomy as contingent rather than inherent to advanced nursing practice
   C. Do not address patient safety concerns
   D. Are too focused on rural populations

4. **Which statement best describes the "shared clinical space" discussed in the chapter?**
   A. NPs and physicians sharing office space to reduce costs
   B. The overlapping diagnostic and therapeutic authority exercised by NPs and physicians
   C. Interprofessional team meetings
   D. Collaborative practice agreements required by law

5. **The primary purpose of this book is to:**
   A. Advocate for regulatory changes expanding NP scope
   B. Prove NPs are equivalent to physicians
   C. Provide a nursing-centered theoretical framework explaining autonomous practice
   D. Replace existing nursing theories

6. **When the chapter discusses "internalized uncertainty," it refers to:**
   A. Students' anxiety about certification exams
   B. NPs questioning their clinical skills
   C. NPs experiencing doubt about professional legitimacy despite bearing full responsibility
   D. Uncertainty about which specialty to choose

7. **The central problem of autonomous practice, according to this chapter, is:**
   A. Whether NPs are capable of independent clinical authority
   B. How autonomous authority is understood
   C. Whether regulations should be changed
   D. How to increase NP salaries

8. **Nursopathic medicine applies specifically to:**
   A. All nursing practice from RN through DNP
   B. Nurse practitioner practice at the APRN level
   C. Only psychiatric-mental health NPs
   D. Nurse educators and administrators

9. **The term "medicine" in this book refers to:**
   A. The exclusive practice of physicians
   B. The practice domain of diagnosing and treating disease
   C. Only allopathic medical practice
   D. Hospital-based care

10. **The book's focus on "how" rather than "whether" NPs practice autonomously reflects:**
    A. Assumption that autonomy already exists and needs explanation
    B. Avoidance of controversial topics
    C. Agreement with restrictive practice models
    D. Focus on regulatory advocacy

CASE-BASED APPLICATION QUESTIONS

Case Scenario 1:

Maria is a newly graduated FNP working in a state with full practice authority. She independently diagnoses and treats patients, prescribes medications, and manages chronic conditions. However, when asked by a patient how her practice differs from the physician in the next exam room, she struggles to articulate an answer beyond "I'm a nurse practitioner, not a doctor."

Questions:

- How does Maria's situation illustrate the "conceptual gap" described in Chapter 1?
- What consequences of conceptual ambiguity might Maria experience, according to the chapter?

- How would the nursopathic medicine framework help Maria respond to the patient's question?

Case Scenario 2:

A state nursing association is preparing testimony for a legislative hearing on full practice authority. They have compiled extensive outcome data showing NP care is safe and effective. However, legislators still express confusion about "what exactly NPs do that's different from physicians" and "whether this is really nursing or medicine."

Questions:

- Why might outcome data alone be insufficient to address legislators' concerns, based on this chapter?
- What conceptual problem do the legislators' questions reveal?
- How could the nursopathic medicine framework strengthen the testimony?

TRUE/FALSE SELF-ASSESSMENT

1. ______ The conceptual gap exists because NPs lack clinical competence.
2. ______ Autonomous practice means NPs never collaborate with physicians.
3. ______ Historical narratives about NP practice (access, collaboration) are accurate but insufficient for explaining contemporary autonomous practice.
4. ______ Nursopathic medicine applies to both RN and NP practice.
5. ______ Medicine, as used in this book, refers to the practice domain of diagnosing and treating disease.

See Appendix B for complete answers and rationales.

CHAPTER 2

THE HISTORICAL DEVELOPMENT OF THE NURSE PRACTITIONER ROLE

LEARNING OBJECTIVES

Upon completing this chapter, students will be able to:

Trace the evolution of the nurse practitioner role from its mid-20th century origins to contemporary practice.

Explain how Hildegard Peplau's theoretical work in psychiatric nursing established precedent for autonomous advanced practice.

Describe the key principles from Peplau's work that foreshadowed nursopathic medicine (independent therapeutic authority, graduate-level preparation, role expansion without abandonment).

Compare the historical framing of NP practice (collaboration, access, delegation) with contemporary practice realities.

Analyze why historical justification alone is insufficient for explaining current autonomous practice.

Identify parallel developments in international contexts (UK, Canada, Australia, New Zealand).

Evaluate the limits of history as a foundation for professional theory, and explain what a forward-looking conceptual framework must provide that history cannot.

CRITICAL THINKING QUESTIONS

Historical Analysis: How did Peplau's argument that psychiatric nurses practicing psychotherapy were "extending nursing" rather than "becoming psychologists" establish a precedent for contemporary NP practice? What are the parallels?

Comparison: Compare the challenges Peplau faced in explaining autonomous psychiatric nursing in the 1950s with the challenges this book addresses for contemporary NPs. What has changed? What remains the same?

Evaluation: The chapter states that "history explains how the role developed, but not how it currently functions as an autonomous clinical profession." Do you agree or disagree? Defend your position.

Application: Choose one international context mentioned (Canada, UK, Australia, New Zealand). How did the NP or advanced practice nursing role develop there, and what similarities or differences do you find compared to the U.S. trajectory?

Synthesis: If you were designing a new advanced practice nursing role today (rather than inheriting the historical NP model), what would you do differently based on lessons from this chapter?

Reflection: How does learning about Peplau's pioneering work change your understanding of what it means to practice autonomously as a nurse? What does it mean to you to practice a role that thought leaders had to argue for and defend?

Critical Thinking: The chapter suggests that grounding NP legitimacy primarily in "access, collaboration, or equivalence arguments" reinforces the perception that autonomy is contingent rather than inherent. Explain this argument and evaluate whether you find it convincing.

1. THEORETICAL FOUNDATIONS: PEPLAU AND THE SEEDS OF ADVANCED PRACTICE

Before the nurse practitioner role emerged in the 1960s, theoretical foundations were being established that would eventually support autonomous practice. Hildegard Peplau's groundbreaking work in psychiatric nursing provided early evidence that nursing could integrate diagnostic reasoning and therapeutic intervention within a nursing framework, without becoming something other than nursing (Peplau, 1952).

2. PEPLAU'S CONTRIBUTION TO AUTONOMOUS PRACTICE THEORY

Hildegard Peplau (1909-1999), often called the "mother of psychiatric nursing," developed the first systematic theory of nursing practice that explicitly addressed the therapeutic role of nurses. Her *Interpersonal Relations in Nursing* (1952) described nursing as an interpersonal process in which nurses function as therapeutic agents, not merely as assistants to physicians (Peplau, 1952).

Several aspects of Peplau's work foreshadowed the theoretical needs that nursopathic medicine now addresses:

2.1 Independent Therapeutic Authority

Peplau described nurses engaging in psychotherapy, a practice traditionally reserved for physicians and psychologists. She argued that nurses, through their unique relational approach, could practice psychotherapy independently within a nursing framework. This was an early articulation of how nursing could incorporate activities from other disciplines while remaining distinctly nursing.

2.2 Assessment and Diagnosis

Peplau's model included thorough patient assessment and identification of nursing diagnoses based on interpersonal dynamics and psychological processes. While her language differed from medical diagnosis, her framework demonstrated that nurses engage in systematic diagnostic reasoning as part of therapeutic practice.

2.3 Phases of Practice

Peplau described nursing practice as occurring in phases (orientation, identification, exploitation, resolution), each requiring different nursing interventions. This phase-based model anticipated later frameworks (including nursopathic medicine's domains) that organize nursing practice by function rather than task (Peplau, 1952).

2.4 Graduate-Level Preparation

Peplau insisted that advanced psychiatric nursing required master's-level education, including supervised clinical practice in psychotherapy. She recognized that autonomous therapeutic practice required specialized preparation beyond basic nursing education. A principle that became foundational to all advanced practice nursing (NCSBN, 2008; AACN, 2021).

2.5 Role Expansion Without Role Abandonment

Critically, Peplau argued that nurses practicing psychotherapy were not abandoning nursing for psychology or psychiatry. They were extending nursing through application of psychological knowledge within a nursing framework centered on therapeutic relationships (Peplau, 1997; Delaney & Shattell, 2013). This principle (integration without professional abandonment) directly informs nursopathic medicine's claim that nurse practitioners practice medicine through nursing.

3. HISTORICAL SIGNIFICANCE FOR AUTONOMOUS PRACTICE

Peplau's work established several precedents relevant to contemporary nurse practitioner practice:

- **Theoretical legitimacy** for nursing roles that include activities traditionally associated with other professions
- **Recognition** that advanced practice requires graduate-level education and specialized training
- **Framework** for understanding how nursing can integrate knowledge from other disciplines while maintaining professional identity
- **Advocacy** for autonomous nursing practice based on nursing expertise, not physician delegation

While Peplau's focus was psychiatric nursing, her theoretical contributions created conceptual space for advanced practice nursing more broadly. She demonstrated that nursing theory could account for independent therapeutic authority grounded in nursing's distinct epistemology and relational focus.

4. FROM PEPLAU TO NURSE PRACTITIONERS

The nurse practitioner role that emerged in the 1960s developed along a different trajectory (focused initially on primary care and physical health rather than mental health) but faced similar conceptual challenges. Just as Peplau had to explain how nurses practicing psychotherapy remained nurses, later theorists would need to explain how nurse practitioners diagnosing and treating illness remained nurses.

Peplau's framework provided theoretical precedent but not a complete model. Her work was specific to psychiatric nursing and did not address the breadth of medical decision-making that nurse practitioners would eventually assume. Nevertheless, her insistence that advanced nursing practice could be both autonomous and distinctly nursing established a foundation upon which later advanced practice roles could build.

The historical trajectory from Peplau's psychiatric nursing theory to the nurse practitioner role reveals a consistent pattern: nursing has repeatedly expanded its scope to include activities requiring independent clinical judgment, therapeutic authority, and integration of biomedical knowledge—always through a nursing framework rather than by adopting another profession's identity.

This pattern suggests that nursopathic medicine does not represent a radical departure from nursing's evolution, but rather a continuation of theoretical development that began decades before the first nurse practitioner programs.

5. ORIGINS IN PRACTICAL NEED

The nurse practitioner role emerged in the mid-twentieth century in response to practical needs within the healthcare system. Early programs were designed to expand access to care, particularly in primary care and underserved settings. These roles were initially framed as extensions of nursing practice, emphasizing health promotion, disease prevention, and continuity of care. Medical diagnosis and treatment were present but often described as delegated or supervised functions.

6. EVOLUTION TOWARD AUTONOMY

As the role evolved, nurse practitioners increasingly assumed responsibility for comprehensive patient care. Educational standards expanded, certification processes formalized, and regulatory frameworks developed to reflect growing clinical authority. Over time, nurse practitioners moved from settings defined by physician oversight to environments characterized by independent practice, including full practice authority in many jurisdictions.

7. THE LIMITS OF HISTORICAL NARRATIVE

Despite these changes, much of the historical narrative surrounding nurse practitioners has remained anchored in origin stories of collaboration and access. While historically accurate, this framing has limited explanatory power for contemporary practice. History explains how the role developed, but not how it currently functions as an autonomous clinical profession.

As nurse practitioner practice expanded, education increasingly emphasized diagnostic reasoning, pharmacology, and disease management alongside nursing theory. However, nursing's conceptual frameworks did not evolve in parallel to explain how these medical functions were integrated into nursing practice. Instead, autonomy was often justified pragmatically (through workforce needs, outcome data, or legal authority) rather than theoretically.

8. THE PROBLEM OF CONTINGENT LEGITIMACY

This reliance on historical justification has unintentionally reinforced the perception that nurse practitioner autonomy is contingent rather than inherent. By grounding legitimacy primarily in access, collaboration, or equivalence arguments, the profession has left unanswered the deeper question of how advanced nursing practice encompasses medical diagnosis and treatment as a distinct professional activity.

The consequences of this gap are not merely academic. In a media environment where scope of practice debates are fought in headlines and social media threads—where terms like "scope creep," "dangerous," and "unqualified" echo across platforms and drown out substantive professional discourse. A profession without a clear theoretical account of its own authority is vulnerable. Nurse practitioners who cannot articulate the theoretical basis of their autonomous practice are left relying on the same historical and pragmatic arguments that the opposition has learned to contest. The echo chamber grows louder, and the professional voice that should answer it goes unheard.

I did not write this book to advocate for scope expansion, though I believe such expansion is just. I wrote it because a voice is needed to pierce those echoes: a theoretical account grounded in nursing itself that explains, from the inside, what autonomous NP practice is and why it is coherent. That is what Peplau understood about psychiatric nursing in the 1950s. It is what nursopathic medicine attempts to provide now.

9. MOVING BEYOND HISTORY

Understanding this historical trajectory is essential, not to re-litigate past debates, but to recognize the limits of history as a foundation for theory. Autonomous practice today cannot be fully explained by the circumstances that gave rise to the nurse practitioner role. It requires a forward-looking model that reflects the realities of modern practice and provides conceptual clarity for the future.

10. INTERNATIONAL EMERGENCE OF ADVANCED PRACTICE NURSING

While this chapter has focused on U.S. history, advanced practice nursing roles emerged internationally through parallel and sometimes interconnected developments. The United Kingdom, Canada, Australia, and New Zealand developed nurse practitioner or advanced nurse practitioner roles beginning in the 1960s-1990s, often influenced by U.S. models but adapted to their respective healthcare systems (Bryant-Lukosius & DiCenso, 2004; Kleinpell et al., 2014; Delamaire & Lafortune, 2010).

These international developments faced similar conceptual challenges: defining scope, establishing educational standards, negotiating relationships with medicine, and articulating professional identity. The global emergence of autonomous advanced practice nursing suggests that nursopathic medicine addresses universal needs within nursing's evolution rather than U.S.-specific circumstances. Despite different regulatory frameworks and titles (Advanced Nurse Practitioner in the UK, Nurse Practitioner in Canada and Australia), these roles share common features: graduate-level education, autonomous clinical decision-making, diagnostic and prescriptive authority, and responsibility for patient outcomes.

The international trajectory parallels the U.S. experience: practical workforce needs drove role creation, but theoretical frameworks lagged behind practice realities. Just as U.S. nurse practitioners required conceptual clarity beyond historical justification, international advanced practice nurses need frameworks that explain how autonomous medical practice integrates with nursing identity across diverse healthcare systems.

Clinical Reflction: A Voice Lost in Echoes

We live in a tumultuous world. Conflict and discord dominate the news cycle and saturate social media. For nurse practitioners, this environment has a specific texture: the scope of practice debate plays out not in measured professional discourse but in the language of alarm. Terms like "scope creep," "dangerous," and "unqualified" echo across platforms, amplified by algorithms that reward provocation over precision. The echo chamber does not argue. It accumulates. And a professional voice that cannot match its volume or its confidence can find itself drowned out entirely.

I did not write this book to advocate for scope expansion, though I believe such expansion is just. I wrote it because the echo needed an answer that the profession had not yet fully provided: not a louder argument, but a deeper one. A theoretical account, grounded in nursing itself, that explains from the inside what autonomous nurse practitioner practice is and why it is coherent. History alone cannot provide that account. Workforce data cannot provide it. Outcome studies, as important as they are, cannot provide it either. What was missing was a nursing-centered framework that explains not just that NPs practice autonomously, but how that practice functions as nursing.

Peplau understood this. In the 1950s, when psychiatric nurses began practicing psychotherapy, they encountered their own version of the echo chamber: the claim that what they were doing was not nursing, that they were practicing psychology without proper credentials, that their authority was derivative and their identity confused. Peplau's answer was not to abandon the claim to autonomous practice. It was to provide the theoretical structure that explained how psychotherapy, practiced by nurses within a nursing relational framework, was an extension of nursing rather than a departure from it. She gave the profession a voice that could answer the criticism on its own terms.

Nursing thought leaders like Peplau did not simply advance the profession; they gave it the theoretical language needed to defend itself. Every framework this book builds on, every conceptual tool it uses to explain autonomous NP practice, rests on foundations they laid. This book is, in that sense, an act of gratitude as much as an act of theory. The logical structure at the heart of nursopathic medicine, that nurse practitioners practicing medicine are extending nursing rather than abandoning it, just as psychiatric nurses practicing psychotherapy were extending nursing rather than becoming psychologists—is an argument Peplau made first, in a different context, more than seventy years ago. The work continues because of the giants that came first.

I am grateful for every nursing thought leader who paved the way for NPs to practice and exercise autonomous nursing judgment. Their work was not simply historical; it was an act of professional courage in an environment that questioned whether their authority was legitimate. The echoes they faced were different in form but not in substance from the ones NPs encounter today. What they left behind was not just precedent. It was a demonstration that the professional voice can, with sufficient theoretical grounding, pierce the noise.

That is what this book attempts to do. Not to win a debate, but to provide the grounding that makes a coherent answer possible.

CHAPTER SUMMARY

The nurse practitioner role evolved from practical needs to autonomous clinical authority through expanding education, regulation, and practice scope. However, historical narratives of collaboration and access, while accurate, provide insufficient theoretical foundation for contemporary autonomous practice. Peplau's theoretical contribution—demonstrating that nurses could practice psychotherapy as an extension of nursing rather than an abandonment of it—established the logical precedent that nursopathic medicine now applies to the full scope of NP autonomous practice. A forward-looking conceptual framework is needed to explain how nurse practitioners currently function as independent clinicians within nursing's professional identity, and to give the profession a theoretical voice capable of answering the echoes that contemporary scope debates produce.

CHAPTER 2
PRACTICE QUESTIONS

MULTIPLE CHOICE QUESTIONS

1. **Hildegard Peplau's primary contribution to autonomous practice theory was:**
   A. Creating the first NP program
   B. Demonstrating that nurses could practice psychotherapy independently within a nursing framework, extending nursing rather than abandoning it
   C. Proving NPs are equivalent to physicians
   D. Developing prescriptive authority for nurses

2. **Peplau's work established which precedent relevant to contemporary NP practice?**
   A. Nurses should replace psychologists
   B. Nursing can integrate activities from other disciplines while maintaining professional identity
   C. Graduate education is unnecessary for advanced practice
   D. Collaboration always requires physician oversight

3. **Peplau insisted that advanced psychiatric nursing required:**
   A. Medical school training
   B. Physician supervision
   C. Master's-level education including supervised clinical practice
   D. Only certification, not a graduate degree

4. **Peplau's principle of "role expansion without role abandonment" means:**
   A. Nurses can practice any healthcare role
   B. Nurses practicing psychotherapy were extending nursing, not becoming psychologists
   C. Nurses must abandon traditional nursing when advancing
   D. Role expansion requires physician delegation

5. **The chapter argues that grounding NP legitimacy primarily in access, collaboration, or equivalence arguments:**
   A. Is the most effective approach to scope advocacy
   B. Reinforces the perception that autonomy is contingent rather than inherent
   C. Addresses all conceptual concerns about NP practice
   D. Is required by regulatory bodies

6. **The chapter states that historical narratives have limited explanatory power for contemporary practice because:**
   A. History is inaccurate
   B. The NP role hasn't changed since inception
   C. History explains how the role developed, not how it currently functions as an autonomous clinical profession
   D. Historical justifications are no longer legal

7. **As NP practice evolved, educational standards:**
   A. Remained at certificate level
   B. Expanded to include diagnostic reasoning, pharmacology, and disease management alongside nursing theory
   C. Decreased in rigor
   D. Focused exclusively on wellness and prevention

8. **The chapter's discussion of "echoes" in the scope of practice debate refers to:**
   A. The repetition of NP outcome data across journals
   B. The amplification of terms like "scope creep" and "dangerous" in media and social platforms that drown out substantive professional discourse
   C. Peplau's influence on successive nursing theorists
   D. International regulatory variation

9. **Peplau's Interpersonal Relations in Nursing was published in:**
   A. 1942 B. 1952
   C. 1962 D. 1972

10. **International development of advanced practice nursing suggests:**
    A. Only the US has autonomous NPs
    B. Nursopathic medicine addresses universal needs within nursing's evolution, not U.S.-specific circumstances
    C. Other countries have fully resolved the conceptual challenges this book addresses
    D. International advanced practice roles are fundamentally different from U.S. NP practices

CASE-BASED APPLICATION QUESTIONS

Case Scenario 1:

Dr. Sarah Thompson, a PMHNP, is challenged by a psychologist colleague who says, "You're just doing what we do—that's not nursing, that's psychology." Sarah remembers reading about Peplau's work and how psychiatric nurses established precedent for autonomous therapeutic practice.

Questions:

- How did Peplau address similar challenges in the 1950s regarding psychiatric nurses practicing psychotherapy?

- What parallel exists between Peplau's situation and contemporary NP practice?
- How does the "echoes" problem described in the clinical reflection relate to the committee's framing of the debate?

Case Scenario 2:

A legislative committee is debating full practice authority for NPs. Proponents cite the 60+ year history of NPs providing safe, effective care. However, the committee remains unconvinced, stating "We understand the history, but we still don't understand what makes this nursing versus medicine."

Questions:

- Why is historical justification insufficient to address the committee's concern?
- What conceptual question are legislators asking that history alone cannot answer?
- What does the chapter suggest is needed beyond historical narrative?

TRUE/FALSE SELF-ASSESSMENT

1. ______ Peplau is called the "mother of psychiatric nursing."
2. ______ The NP role emerged primarily to address physician shortages in rural areas.
3. ______ Peplau demonstrated that graduate-level education was necessary for autonomous therapeutic practice.
4. ______ The chapter argues that history explains how the NP role developed but not how it currently functions as an autonomous clinical profession.
5. ______ Peplau's framework provided a complete and sufficient model for contemporary NP practice.

See Appendix B for complete answers and rationales.

CHAPTER 3

DEFINING NURSOPATHIC MEDICINE

LEARNING OBJECTIVES

Upon completing this chapter, students will be able to:

Define nursopathic medicine and explain its purpose as a conceptual framework.

Distinguish between medicine as a practice domain and "the practice of medicine" as a legal/regulatory term.

Explain how medicine can be approached through different professional frameworks (allopathic, osteopathic, nursopathic).

Articulate what makes nursopathic medicine distinctly "nursing" despite including medical diagnosis and treatment.

Describe the five defining features of nursopathic medicine (autonomous authority, evidence-based practice, integrated assessment, accountability).

Compare nursopathic medicine to allopathic and osteopathic medicine, identifying similarities and differences.

Evaluate why using the term "medicine" is necessary for conceptual clarity rather than obscuring what NPs do.

Apply the concept that nursopathic medicine applies only to NP practice, not RN practice.

CRITICAL THINKING QUESTIONS

Conceptual Analysis: The chapter defines medicine as a "practice domain" rather than exclusive to any profession. How does this definition challenge or support your previous understanding of what "practicing medicine" means?

Professional Identity: If NPs diagnose, prescribe, and treat illness (activities associated with medicine), what specifically makes them nurses rather than physicians? Use the chapter's framework to construct your answer.

Evaluation: Some might argue that using the term "nursopathic medicine" creates confusion or challenges physician scope. Others argue it creates necessary clarity. Which position do you find more compelling and why?

Application: Consider a family nurse practitioner managing a patient with diabetes. How would you explain that they are practicing "nursopathic medicine" rather than "allopathic medicine" even though the clinical activities may look similar?

Integration: The chapter states nursopathic medicine represents integration of nursing (identity, ethics, epistemology) + medicine (diagnosis, treatment, biomedical science) + autonomous practice. Why is this integration rather than "hybridization or role blurring"?

Reflection: A patient calls you "doctor" during a clinical encounter. Using the framework from this chapter, explain what that moment reveals about the patient's perception of what you are doing—and why it is neither a mistake nor a confusion to be corrected.

Professional Identity: Does defining nurse practitioner practice as "nursopathic medicine" strengthen or weaken nursing's professional identity? Defend your position with specific reasoning.

1. INTRODUCTION: A CONCEPTUAL FRAMEWORK

Nursopathic medicine is proposed in this text as a conceptual framework that explains how nurse practitioners practice medicine autonomously through advanced nursing practice. It is not a claim of new licensure, title, or statutory authority, but a theory intended to clarify existing clinical realities. By defining nursopathic medicine, this chapter seeks to provide nursing with an internally coherent explanation for the integration of medical diagnosis and treatment within its highest level of practice.

2. SCOPE OF APPLICATION

Nursopathic medicine applies specifically to nurse practitioner practice at the advanced practice registered nurse (APRN) level, the role in which autonomous diagnostic and therapeutic decision-making is the defining feature of clinical activity. Certified nurse midwives engage in this diagnostic-therapeutic model within their reproductive and women's health scope, and the framework applies within that context. Certified registered nurse anesthetists and clinical nurse specialists operate under fundamentally different practice models and are therefore outside the scope of this framework—not because their practice is less significant, but because the framework is built around a specific practice model that does not describe their work. It does not describe registered nursing practice, which operates under a different scope of practice, authority structure, and model of accountability. The framework addresses doctoral-level or master's-level prepared nurse practitioners who hold national certification and practice with independent diagnostic and prescriptive authority (NCSBN, 2008).

3. MEDICINE AS PRACTICE DOMAIN, NOT PROFESSIONAL IDENTITY

Before articulating how nursopathic medicine functions as a framework, it is necessary to clarify what is meant by "medicine" within this text. The term carries multiple meanings in contemporary healthcare, and precision is required to avoid confusion or misinterpretation.

4. DEFINING MEDICINE

Medicine, as used in nursopathic medicine, refers to the systematic body of knowledge and clinical practice concerned with:

- The diagnosis of disease and pathophysiological processes
- The therapeutic management of illness through pharmacologic and procedural interventions

- The prevention of disease through risk assessment and clinical intervention
- The longitudinal management of chronic conditions
- The application of biomedical science to patient care

This definition describes medicine as a practice domain (a field of knowledge and action) rather than as the exclusive property of any single profession. Medicine, in this sense, encompasses the activities of assessing, diagnosing, treating, and managing human health conditions through application of biomedical science.

5. MEDICINE DISTINGUISHED FROM "THE PRACTICE OF MEDICINE"

It is essential to distinguish between medicine as a practice domain, which is what this book describes, and "the practice of medicine" as a legal and regulatory term. State medical practice acts often define "the practice of medicine" as activities reserved for physicians. These legal definitions exist to regulate professional boundaries and protect public safety. However, legal definitions of professional scope do not determine the conceptual boundaries of clinical knowledge or practice domains.

Many healthcare professions engage in activities that involve medical knowledge and medical decision-making (including diagnosis, treatment, and prescribing) without claiming to practice "medicine" in the physician-specific legal sense. Advanced practice registered nurses, including nurse practitioners, are among these professions (Hamric et al., 2014).

6. MEDICINE THROUGH MULTIPLE PROFESSIONAL LENSES

Medicine as a practice domain can be approached through different professional frameworks:

- **Allopathic Medicine (MD)**: Medicine practiced through the professional tradition, education, and licensure of allopathic physicians, grounded in biomedical science and clinical training within medical schools and residency programs.

- **Osteopathic Medicine (DO):** Medicine practiced through the osteopathic professional tradition, emphasizing whole-person and manipulative approaches alongside biomedical science.
- **Nursopathic Medicine (NP):** Medicine practiced through the professional tradition, education, and licensure of nurse practitioners, grounded in nursing epistemology, biomedical science, and advanced nursing judgment.

Each profession brings its distinct values, education, and orientation to the practice domain of medicine. The activities (diagnosing, prescribing, treating) may overlap, but the professional framework through which they are understood, justified, and executed differs.

7. WHAT MAKES NURSOPATHIC MEDICINE "NURSING"

If nurse practitioners engage in diagnosis, treatment, and prescribing (activities traditionally associated with medicine) what makes nursopathic medicine distinctly "nursing"?

The answer lies in **professional framework, not task performance:**

- **Educational Foundation:** Nurse practitioners are educated within nursing programs, by nursing faculty, using nursing frameworks. Even when learning pathophysiology and pharmacology, the application is filtered through nursing's patient-centered, patient-centered orientation.
- **Epistemological Grounding:** Nursopathic medicine reflects nursing's ways of knowing, emphasizing context, relationships, functional outcomes, and the patient's lived experience alongside biomedical data (Carper, 1978; Meleis, 2018).
- **Ethical Framework:** Clinical decisions are guided by nursing ethics, including advocacy, patient empowerment, and attention to social determinants of health (ANA, 2015; Grace, 2018).

- **Professional Identity:** Nurse practitioners identify as nurses, are accountable to nursing regulatory bodies, and practice within nursing's scope, even when that scope includes medical diagnosis and treatment.
- **Licensure and Regulation:** Authority to diagnose and prescribe derives from nursing licensure (advanced practice registered nurse), not medical licensure.

Nursopathic medicine does not claim that nurse practitioners are physicians or that they practice allopathic or osteopathic medicine. It claims that they engage in medical practice as nurse practitioners, through a nursing framework.

This principle echoes Peplau's earlier work in psychiatric nursing, where she demonstrated that nurses could practice psychotherapy (an activity associated with other professions) while remaining grounded in nursing's therapeutic and relational orientation (Peplau, 1952; Peplau, 1997). Just as Peplau showed that psychiatric nurses practicing psychotherapy were extending nursing rather than abandoning it, nursopathic medicine argues that nurse practitioners practicing medicine are operating within an expanded nursing scope, not adopting physician identity.

8. WHY "MEDICINE" LANGUAGE MATTERS

Some may question why this framework uses the term "medicine" at all. Why not simply describe nurse practitioner practice as "advanced nursing practice" without reference to medicine?

The reason is clarity and honesty. Nurse practitioners:

- Generate differential diagnoses
- Order and interpret diagnostic tests
- Prescribe medications and treatments
- Manage acute and chronic illnesses
- Assume responsibility for clinical outcomes

These activities constitute medical practice in the descriptive sense, they involve applying biomedical knowledge to diagnose and treat disease. To avoid the language of medicine would obscure what nurse practitioners actually do and perpetuate the conceptual ambiguity this book seeks to resolve.

The claim is not that all nursing involves medicine, nor that medicine encompasses all of nursing. Rather, **at the advanced practice level, nursing integrates medical practice within its scope.** This integration occurs through nursing's professional lens, not by adopting physician identity or relinquishing nursing values.

9. NURSOPATHIC MEDICINE AS INTEGRATION

Nursopathic medicine, then, represents the integration of:

- **Nursing** (professional identity, education, ethics, epistemology)
- **Medicine** (diagnosis, treatment, biomedical science, therapeutic management)
- **Autonomous practice** (independent authority and accountability within scope)

This integration is not hybridization or role blurring. It is the recognition that advanced nursing practice, at the nurse practitioner level, includes medical decision-making as an inherent component, practiced through nursing, accountable to nursing standards, and serving nursing's patient-centered mission.

The five domains that follow (Acute Care, Chronic Care, Preventative Care, Interdisciplinary Care, and Specialty Care) describe how this integrated practice functions across the full scope of nurse practitioner responsibility.

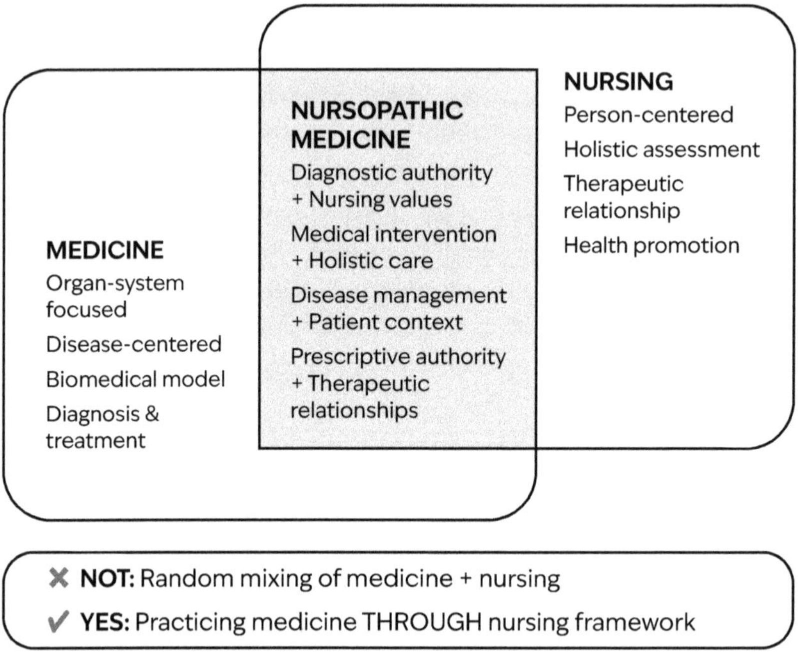

Figure 3.1. Nursopathic Medicine: Integration, Not Hybridization.

10. CORE RECOGNITION: MEDICINE WITHIN NURSING

At its core, nursopathic medicine recognizes that nurse practitioners engage in the full spectrum of clinical decision-making traditionally associated with medical care, including diagnostic evaluation, therapeutic planning, and longitudinal management of illness. What distinguishes this practice is not the tasks performed, but the professional framework through which those tasks are understood, justified, and executed. Nursopathic medicine locates medical practice firmly within nursing's epistemology, ethics, and accountability structures.

11. DISTINCTION FROM OTHER MEDICAL PRACTICE MODELS

Unlike allopathic or osteopathic medicine, which define practice through professional lineage and disciplinary tradition, nursopathic medicine is defined by its orientation to care. Clinical authority arises from nursing education, certification, and licensure, and is exercised within a framework that prioritizes patient context, functional outcomes, and continuity across the lifespan. The practice of medicine is not adopted from another profession, but emerges naturally from advanced nursing judgment.

12. NOT ROLE SUBSTITUTION

Defining nursopathic medicine also requires distinguishing it from role substitution or professional overlap. Nursopathic medicine does not position nurse practitioners as replacements for physicians, nor does it rely on equivalence arguments to justify autonomy. Instead, it asserts that nurse practitioners practice medicine as nurse practitioners, guided by nursing values and informed by biomedical science. This distinction is critical for maintaining professional clarity and avoiding adversarial framing.

13. DEFINING FEATURES

The defining features of nursopathic medicine include autonomous clinical authority, evidence-based decision-making (Melnyk & Fineout-Overholt, 2019), holistic patient assessment, and accountability for outcomes. Autonomy within this model is not isolationist; it is exercised within interdisciplinary systems of care. Collaboration is assumed, expected, and valued (IPEC, 2016), but it does not negate independent responsibility for clinical decisions within scope.

14. PROVIDING PROFESSIONAL LANGUAGE

By articulating nursopathic medicine as a defined practice model, nursing gains a language to describe what nurse practitioners already do. This definition provides conceptual stability, allowing autonomous practice to be understood as a legitimate, enduring, and professionally grounded mode of advanced nursing practice rather than an exception or expansion.

Clinical Reflection: "Are You My Doctor?"

It happens regularly. A patient, often one I have been managing for months, turns to me at the end of an encounter and says: "Thank you, doctor." Sometimes it is a new patient who has just experienced their first appointment with me and did not register the NP after my name. Sometimes it is a patient who knows exactly what I am and calls me doctor anyway, because in their mind, in that room, that is what they see.

For a long time, I did not know how to hold that moment. The technically correct response is to gently clarify: "I'm actually a nurse practitioner, not a physician." And I offer that clarification. But I noticed something about the way patients receive it. They are not embarrassed. They do not feel they made an error. They nod, sometimes smile, and the word "doctor" still lingers in the room like something true that has been re-labeled but not changed. They perceived something real. The title was imprecise. The perception was not.

What patients perceive when they call a nurse practitioner "doctor" is autonomous clinical authority being exercised on their behalf. They experience a clinician who is asking them questions, examining them, ordering tests, making a diagnosis, writing a prescription, and assuming responsibility for what happens next. They do not have a word for it that fits. "Nurse" does not capture it because their understanding of nurses, however incomplete, does not include the person who authors their care plan. "Doctor" is the closest word they have. They reach for it because it is the only available language for what they are experiencing. The conceptual gap is not in the patient. It is in the professional vocabulary available to describe what nurse practitioners actually do.

This is exactly the problem nursopathic medicine is designed to resolve. Without a framework that explains how NPs practice medicine through nursing, that moment of misidentification has no professional answer. The NP corrects the title but cannot fully explain the practice. And in the absence of that explanation, something more corrosive can take hold: the clinician begins to wonder whether the patient's instinct was somehow more accurate than the credential. If what I do looks like medicine, feels like medicine to the patient, and requires the same diagnostic and therapeutic authority as medicine—am I really practicing nursing? The question, unanswered, becomes imposter syndrome. The ambiguity does not stay academic. It gets internalized.

Nursopathic medicine resolves this not by changing what nurse practitioners do, but by providing the language to understand it. The patient who calls me doctor is perceiving nursopathic medicine. They are seeing clinical authority exercised through a nursing framework, one characterized by relational attention, whole-person orientation, and the continuity of care that nursing brings, and they are recognizing it as autonomous clinical practice. They are right. The framework this chapter defines gives that recognition a name, a theoretical basis, and a professional home. It allows the NP to say, with clarity and without apology: what you are experiencing is nursopathic medicine. It is medicine practiced through nursing. It is both, fully, at once.

The imposter syndrome that affects so many nurse practitioners is not a personal failing. It is a predictable consequence of practicing with authority that the profession has not yet fully articulated. When the clinical identity is clear and a framework exists that explains what autonomous NP practice is and why it is coherent, the patient who calls you doctor is no longer a source of anxiety. The patient becomes evidence. They saw, without being told, what nursopathic medicine is.

CHAPTER SUMMARY

Nursopathic medicine is a conceptual framework explaining how nurse practitioners practice medicine autonomously through advanced nursing practice. It is distinguished from other medical models by its grounding in nursing epistemology, ethics, and patient-centered care. The framework does not claim new authority but provides theoretical clarity for existing practice, offering nursing a professional language for autonomous clinical decision-making. Without this framework, the gap between what nurse practitioners do and how that practice is theoretically explained becomes a source of professional ambiguity—one that patients, who perceive autonomous clinical authority directly, do not share.

CHAPTER 3
PRACTICE QUESTIONS

MULTIPLE CHOICE QUESTIONS

1. **Nursopathic medicine is best defined as:**
   A. A claim for new licensure and statutory authority
   B. A conceptual framework explaining how NPs practice medicine through advanced nursing
   C. A replacement for existing nursing theories
   D. A medical specialty for nurses

2. **The term "medicine" in nursopathic medicine refers to:**
   A. The exclusive practice of physicians
   B. The practice domain of diagnosing, treating, and managing disease
   C. Only allopathic medical practice
   D. Hospital-based care exclusively

3. **Nursopathic medicine applies specifically to:**
   A. All levels of nursing practice
   B. Only psychiatric NPs
   C. Nurse practitioner practice at the APRN level
   D. Nursing students and educators

4. **What distinguishes nursopathic medicine from allopathic medicine?**
   A. NPs use different diagnostic criteria
   B. Professional framework, education, ethics, and licensure grounded in nursing
   C. NPs cannot prescribe medications
   D. There is no distinction

5. **The chapter distinguishes between:**
   A. Good nurses and bad nurses
   B. Medicine as a practice domain vs. "the practice of medicine" as legal terminology
   C. Primary care and specialty care
   D. NPs and PAs

6. **Medicine as a practice domain can be approached through which professional frameworks?**
   A. Only allopathic (MD)
   B. Allopathic (MD), osteopathic (DO), and nursopathic (NP)
   C. Any healthcare profession
   D. Only those with medical degrees

7. **What makes nursopathic medicine distinctly "nursing" despite including diagnosis and treatment?**
   A. NPs are supervised by nurses
   B. Educational foundation, epistemological grounding, ethical framework, and professional identity
   C. NPs only treat minor illnesses
   D. Nothing—it's actually medicine, not nursing

8. **When a patient calls a nurse practitioner "doctor," the chapter suggests this reflects:**
   A. Patient confusion about credentials that always requires correction
   B. The patient perceiving autonomous clinical authority being exercised on their behalf—a recognition that is accurate even when the title is not
   C. Evidence that NPs should be reclassified as physicians
   D. A gap in patient health literacy

9. **Using the term "medicine" is necessary for:**
   A. Legal protection
   B. Clarity and honesty about what NPs actually do
   C. Competing with physicians
   D. Marketing purposes

10. **Authority to diagnose and prescribe derives from:**
   A. Physician delegation
   B. Medical licensure
   C. Nursing licensure (APRN)
   D. Hospital privileges

CASE-BASED APPLICATION QUESTIONS

Case Scenario 1:

James, a family NP, is managing a patient with type 2 diabetes, hypertension, and depression. He orders labs, adjusts medications, provides counseling, and coordinates care with a cardiologist. A medical student observes and asks, "If you're diagnosing, prescribing, and treating—isn't that medicine? What makes you a nurse and not a doctor?"

Questions:

- Using the framework from Chapter 3, how would James explain that he's practicing "nursopathic medicine"?
- What specific elements make his practice distinctly nursing despite the medical activities involved?
- How is his practice different from allopathic medicine even when treating the same patient?

Case Scenario 2:

During a hospital credentialing meeting, the medical staff questions whether to grant privileges to acute care NPs, stating "We need to understand if you're practicing medicine or nursing, because the policies are different."

Questions:

- How does this question reflect the conceptual confusion nursopathic medicine addresses?
- What is the correct answer to "medicine or nursing" according to Chapter 3?
- How would you explain that framing the question as either/or is a false dichotomy?

TRUE/FALSE SELF-ASSESSMENT

1. ______ Nursopathic medicine claims new legal authority beyond current NP scope.
2. ______ Medicine as a practice domain is exclusive to physicians.
3. ______ What makes nursopathic medicine "nursing" is the professional framework, not the tasks performed.
4. ______ Nursopathic medicine applies to all nursing levels from RN through DNP.
5. ______ Authority derives from nursing licensure, not medical licensure.

See Appendix B for complete answers and rationales.

CHAPTER 4

METHODS OF CLINICAL REASONING IN NURSOPATHIC MEDICINE

LEARNING OBJECTIVES

Upon completing this chapter, students will be able to:

Name the five methods of clinical reasoning in nursopathic medicine and explain how each corresponds to one of the five practice domains.

Explain how the SOAP note functions as a shared clinical language through which all five reasoning methods operate within a single encounter.

Distinguish the defining clinical question of each reasoning method and articulate what makes it irreplaceable within autonomous practice.

Analyze how Specialty Lens Reasoning differs from the other four methods and explain why it cannot be localized to a specific section of the SOAP note.

Evaluate why concurrent activation of multiple reasoning methods characterizes advanced clinical judgment rather than the sequential application of protocols.

Apply the five reasoning methods to patient scenarios across different specialty contexts, identifying which methods are foregrounded and which are operating in the background.

CRITICAL THINKING QUESTIONS

Analysis: A PMHNP and an FNP both see the same patient for fatigue and insomnia. Their Objective sections look entirely different, yet both are clinically correct. What does this reveal about the nature of clinical observation in autonomous practice, and why would a single standardized Objective format be insufficient across specialties?

Application: Consider a nurse practitioner who practices exclusively in an urgent care setting and argues, "I only do Acute Reasoning—the other four methods don't apply to my work." Using the framework from this chapter, explain why this position reflects a misunderstanding of how the five reasoning methods operate.

Evaluation: The chapter argues that the Assessment section of a SOAP note is "the clinician's most visible act of autonomous reasoning." Do you agree or disagree? What would a weak Assessment reveal about a clinician's reasoning, and what would a strong one demonstrate?

Comparison: Compare Longitudinal Reasoning with single-encounter clinical thinking. What is lost clinically when a patient's care is fragmented across multiple providers who lack a shared longitudinal perspective? How does sustained relationship change what a clinician is able to detect?

Synthesis: The chapter describes Specialty Lens Reasoning as a pervasive filter rather than a localized step. If that is true, what are the obligations of a clinician who encounters a presentation that falls outside their specialty lens, one their training did not equip them to see clearly? How should that recognition be documented and acted upon?

Reflection: The chapter connects Specialty Lens Reasoning to the professional identity uncertainty described in Chapter 1, suggesting that naming the lens reduces the cognitive dissonance behind imposter syndrome. Do you find this argument convincing? Why or why not, and what would it mean clinically if a practitioner internalized that their specialty perspective is a distinct contribution rather than a limitation?

Debate: Some would argue that clinical reasoning is universal, arguing that all clinicians, regardless of profession or specialty, reason the same way and that nursing's claim to distinct methods is theoretical rather than practical. How would you respond to this argument using evidence from this chapter?

1. INTRODUCTION: REASONING AS THE ARCHITECTURE OF PRACTICE

Clinical reasoning is the intellectual engine of autonomous practice. Before the five domains of nursopathic medicine can be understood, and before Acute Care, Chronic Care, Preventative Care, Interdisciplinary Care, and Specialty Care can be practiced with coherence and accountability, the reasoning methods that animate them must be named, distinguished, and understood.

This chapter is a prelude. Its purpose is not to replace the domain chapters that follow but to establish the cognitive architecture that makes them intelligible. Chapters 8 through 12 each explore a domain in full, with detailed clinical case studies and practice questions. This chapter explains how an NP thinks within those domains: what kind of reasoning is active, what clinical question it is answering, and how a single encounter can draw on multiple reasoning methods at once.

Nursopathic medicine identifies five methods of clinical reasoning, each corresponding to one of the five practice domains. Acute Reasoning asks: What is happening right now, and what must I do? Longitudinal Reasoning asks: How has this patient changed over time, and how do I adjust? Anticipatory Reasoning asks: What harm can I foresee and prevent before it happens? Interdisciplinary Reasoning asks: When does another discipline's expertise enhance this patient's care? And Specialty Lens Reasoning asks: How does my specialty context reframe everything I observe?

These five methods do not operate in isolation. They are woven together in every clinical encounter. A practitioner seeing a patient with new-onset chest pain simultaneously engages Acute Reasoning to ask what is happening right now, Longitudinal Reasoning to ask how this compares to prior visits, Anticipatory Reasoning to identify what complications this patient is at risk for, Interdisciplinary Reasoning to determine whether cardiology is needed, and Specialty Lens Reasoning to notice which features her training leads her to prioritize. The skill of autonomous practice lies not in applying each method sequentially, but in holding them simultaneously, knowing which one to foreground in any given moment.

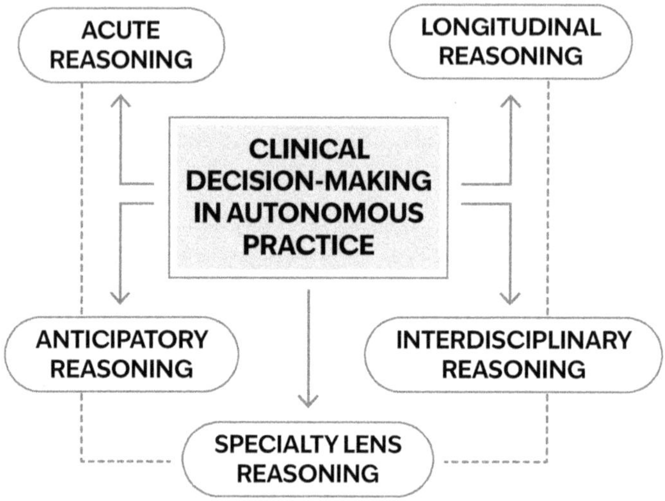

Figure 4.1. Five Methods of Clinical Reasoning in Nursopathic Medicine.

2. THE SOAP NOTE AS A SHARED CLINICAL LANGUAGE

Before examining each reasoning method individually, it is worth establishing the clinical format through which all five are expressed: the SOAP note.

The SOAP note (Subjective, Objective, Assessment, Plan) is the most widely used documentation format in clinical practice. Developed by Lawrence Weed in the late 1960s as a way to impose structured thinking on clinical records (Weed, 1968), it has endured because the structure maps naturally onto how clinicians actually reason. Each section corresponds to a distinct cognitive operation: the Subjective captures what the patient reports; the Objective captures what the clinician observes and measures; the Assessment synthesizes those findings into a working diagnosis and differential; and the Plan specifies what will be done.

Within nursopathic medicine, the SOAP note becomes something more than a documentation requirement. It is the shared clinical language through which all five reasoning methods operate within a single encounter. The Subjective section carries the patient's own account of urgency, trajectory, and risk. The Objective section is where the specialty lens is most visible: a PMHNP and an FNP examining the same patient will each fill the Objective section with entirely different observational data, each one correct for their specialty. The Assessment is where reasoning converges: Acute Reasoning names the working diagnosis, Longitudinal Reasoning asks whether that hypothesis still holds across prior visits, Anticipatory Reasoning stratifies risk, and Interdisciplinary Reasoning determines whether this case exceeds scope. The Plan executes all of it.

What this means in practice is that the Assessment section of a SOAP note is never just a list of diagnoses. It is the clinician's most visible act of autonomous reasoning, the moment where multiple cognitive frameworks converge on a single patient. When a practitioner writes a rigorous Assessment, they are demonstrating that they saw the patient completely, understood the context, weighed the risks, and made a defensible clinical judgment. That is what nursopathic medicine means when it describes the SOAP note as proof of reasoning rather than a form to fill out.

3. ACUTE REASONING

"What is happening right now, and what must I do?"

Corresponding Domain: Acute Care *(Chapter 8)*

Time compression is the defining condition of Acute Reasoning. It activates when information is incomplete and the cost of inaction may be higher than the cost of a provisional decision. It operates in the first minutes of a chest pain evaluation, a psychiatric crisis, a pediatric febrile seizure, or an acute decompensation on an inpatient unit. It is what experienced clinicians draw on when they recognize that a presentation is dangerous before they can fully articulate why.

Clinical reasoning researchers have long distinguished between fast, pattern-based intuition and slower, analytical deliberation: the former recognizes a STEMI on sight while the latter systematically rules out each item on a differential (Kahneman, 2011; Croskerry, 2002). Acute Reasoning draws on both. It begins with pattern recognition: the rapid synthesis of presenting data into a clinical picture that "looks like" something the practitioner has seen before. It continues with probability, ranking diagnoses by likelihood given what is known, and with threshold judgment: is the risk of acting now greater or less than the risk of waiting for more information? And because acute situations evolve, the assessment is never final. Initial interventions generate new data, which refines the picture, which informs the next decision.

Acute Reasoning is not recklessness. The authority to act in acute situations includes the responsibility to recognize limits and initiate appropriate escalation when warranted. A practitioner who cannot distinguish a presentation requiring immediate independent management from one requiring emergency transfer has not mastered Acute Reasoning; they have adopted urgency without structure. Chapter 8 develops this reasoning method in full, with case studies from primary care, psychiatric, and acute inpatient settings, including Maria's STEMI recognition in a community health center and David's psychiatric emergency on an inpatient unit.

4. LONGITUDINAL REASONING

"How has this patient changed over time, and how do I adjust?"

Corresponding Domain: Chronic Care *(Chapter 9)*

Where Acute Reasoning is defined by urgency, Longitudinal Reasoning is defined by time. It unfolds not within a single encounter but across many, tracking patterns, trends, and deviations that become visible only through sustained observation of the same patient.

Longitudinal Reasoning requires the clinician to hold a dynamic mental model of the patient: not just who they are today, but who they were three months ago, what changed, why it changed, and what that trajectory implies about the future. This model is constantly revised as new data arrives. A diagnosis made at visit one is not locked in; it is a working hypothesis subject to revision as the patient's trajectory unfolds (Tanner, 2006). Goals themselves evolve: a HbA1c target appropriate at age 55 may require recalibration at age 75 following a stroke, and recognizing that shift is not deviation from good care but an expression of it.

The episodic model of care, in which each encounter is treated as independent, is the default structure of fragmented healthcare systems. Longitudinal Reasoning is the antidote. It is what allows the nurse practitioner managing a patient over five years to notice the early cognitive changes that an episodic clinician would miss, to recognize that a patient's apparent medication non-compliance is driven by undisclosed depression, and to build the therapeutic relationship that makes difficult conversations about driving restriction or end-of-life planning possible. Chapter 9 demonstrates this through a five-year case study following an AGPCNP and her patient across prediabetes, hypertension, a TIA, and emerging mild cognitive impairment.

5. ANTICIPATORY REASONING

"What harm can I foresee and prevent before it happens?"

Corresponding Domain: Preventative Care *(Chapter 10)*

Anticipatory Reasoning is oriented toward what has not yet happened. While Acute Reasoning asks what is happening now and Longitudinal Reasoning asks how things have changed, Anticipatory Reasoning asks what might occur if the current trajectory continues unchanged.

This is not speculative. Anticipatory Reasoning is grounded in epidemiology, risk stratification, and prevention evidence. It is the capacity to look at a patient's current clinical picture, including labs, lifestyle, genetics, treatment exposures, and psychological state, and project the likely trajectory forward if conditions remain unchanged. A borderline HbA1c, a prehypertensive blood pressure, a moderate PHQ-9 score: none of these are diagnoses today, but each one marks the beginning of a trajectory that Anticipatory Reasoning identifies, stratifies, and acts on before it becomes a crisis.

A common misconception is that Anticipatory Reasoning belongs only to wellness visits and primary care. It does not. A PMHNP monitoring metabolic effects of antipsychotic medications is performing Anticipatory Reasoning. An AGACNP implementing fall prevention protocols in a hospitalized elder is performing Anticipatory Reasoning. An oncology NP addressing chemotherapy-induced peripheral neuropathy before it impairs function is performing Anticipatory Reasoning. Anticipatory Reasoning applies wherever risk exists, which is everywhere clinicians practice. Chapter 10 develops this through a comprehensive wellness case in which an FNP conducts multi-domain risk stratification for a 52-year-old with clustering cardiovascular, metabolic, psychiatric, and sleep-related risks.

6. INTERDISCIPLINARY REASONING

Corresponding Domain: Interdisciplinary Care *(Chapter 11)*

Interdisciplinary Reasoning asks a question about limits: when does another discipline's expertise enhance this patient's care, and when is it essential? It is not a passive acknowledgment that other professions exist; it is an active, ongoing clinical judgment about when, how, and with whom to engage.

The critical distinction in nursopathic medicine is between collaboration and dependency. Interdisciplinary Reasoning produces collaboration: purposeful engagement with other professionals based on clinical indication, with clear accountability retained by the nurse practitioner (IPEC, 2016). Dependency is its opposite: deferring to others reflexively, without clinical rationale, driven by regulatory structure or institutional hierarchy rather than patient need. Recognizing the limits of one's scope and initiating a specialist referral is not a failure of autonomous practice. It is one of autonomous practice's clearest expressions.

This reasoning type appears most explicitly in the Plan section of the SOAP note, but it is seeded throughout. The Subjective section may reveal a social work need or a behavioral concern that exceeds pharmacologic scope. The Assessment must note when a finding requires specialist input. And the Plan must specify the exact type of interdisciplinary engagement (consultation, referral, co-management, or coordination) and what remains under the NP's ongoing management. Chapter 11 develops this through a detailed exploration of NP-MD, NP-PharmD, and other professional interfaces, including a clinical reflection on navigating pharmacist relationships in a telehealth psychiatric practice.

7. SPECIALTY LENS REASONING

"How does my specialty context reframe everything I observe?"

Corresponding Domain: Specialty Care *(Chapter 12)*

Of the five methods, Specialty Lens Reasoning is the most pervasive and the one most often left unnamed. A practitioner's specialty training, population focus, and certification shape every observation, every differential, and every clinical decision (APRN Joint Dialogue Group, 2008). This influence is not situational. It operates from the first sentence the patient speaks.

Every nurse practitioner brings a specialty lens to clinical encounters. The PMHNP sees the same chief complaint differently than the FNP, who sees it differently than the AGACNP, who sees it differently than the pediatric NP. This is not a limitation; it is a feature. The PMHNP examining a patient with fatigue and poor sleep is not running the same mental checklist as the FNP examining the same patient. The PMHNP's Objective section will center on a Mental Status Examination, the primary observational instrument of psychiatric specialty practice. The FNP's Objective section will center on a physical examination, with thyroid palpation, cardiovascular and respiratory findings, and laboratory values. Both clinicians are filling the same SOAP structure with the data their training equips and requires them to gather. The format is universal. The lens is not.

Specialty Lens Reasoning differs from the other four methods in one important way: it does not localize to a specific section of the SOAP note. It filters the entire encounter. It shapes what the clinician asks for in the Subjective, what data they gather in the Objective, how they frame the differential in the Assessment, and which guidelines and interventions appear in the Plan. It explains not just that a PMHNP and an FNP are trained differently, but how that difference manifests in the act of clinical observation itself, note by note, encounter by encounter.

This reasoning method also has a dimension that goes beyond the cognitive. For nurse practitioners who have experienced the professional identity uncertainty described in Chapter 1, the feeling that their authority is not quite legitimate despite objective evidence of competence, Specialty Lens Reasoning offers grounding. The PMHNP does not need to justify seeing psychiatric presentations through a psychiatric lens. That lens is their expertise. It is what they are trained, certified, and licensed to do. Naming it as a defined clinical method affirms that the nurse practitioner's specialty perspective is not a limitation relative to other clinicians. It is a distinct clinical contribution. Chapter 12 develops the formal boundaries of this reasoning method, including the certification requirements, scope alignment, and professional obligations that govern when a specialty lens can be legitimately claimed.

8. THE FIVE REASONING METHODS IN A SINGLE ENCOUNTER

These methods are not sequential. In practice, they operate simultaneously, with the clinician moving fluidly among them in response to the demands of each encounter. The following clinical scenario makes this visible.

Consider a PMHNP conducting a 30-minute follow-up with a 42-year-old patient who has bipolar I disorder, is on lithium and quetiapine, and presents today with fatigue, weight gain, and "not feeling like myself." Specialty Lens Reasoning activates immediately: fatigue and dysphoria in a bipolar patient on lithium raises a psychiatric differential that would not appear on an FNP's initial list: depressive episode, lithium toxicity, quetiapine metabolic effects, hypothyroidism (a known lithium complication), or subclinical hypomania masked by mood stabilization. Acute Reasoning evaluates safety: is there suicidal ideation, and is this a breakthrough episode requiring urgent intervention or hospitalization? Longitudinal Reasoning asks whether this pattern has appeared before, what triggered the last depressive episode, and whether this is the early stage of a familiar trajectory or something new. Anticipatory Reasoning attends to the metabolic picture: weight gain on quetiapine is a known risk, and if the BMI trend and recent labs point toward metabolic syndrome, the time to intervene is now, not after the diagnosis is established. And Interdisciplinary Reasoning evaluates scope: does this patient need a primary care referral for metabolic monitoring, and if lithium levels are elevated, is an internal medicine consult warranted?

All of this happens within the first few minutes of the encounter. The SOAP note the clinician writes will reflect all five reasoning types, even though the patient came in with a complaint that seemed straightforward. This is what autonomous advanced practice looks like from the inside: not the application of protocols, but the concurrent activation of multiple cognitive frameworks, each informing the others, all grounded in specialty-specific knowledge and nursing's commitment to context, relationship, and the patient as a whole person (Carper, 1978; Meleis, 2018).

9. CONCLUSION: REASONING AS PREPARATION FOR THE DOMAINS

These methods are not separate tools to be applied one at a time. They are interwoven cognitive capacities that define what it means to practice autonomously within nursopathic medicine. Chapters 8 through 12 will each develop one reasoning method in full clinical context, placing it within its corresponding practice domain and demonstrating how it functions when the other four are operating alongside it.

The SOAP note, introduced here as the shared clinical language of all five reasoning methods, provides the lens through which the clinical encounters in the chapters that follow should be read. When a nurse practitioner writes a rigorous SOAP note, they are not filling out a form. They are demonstrating autonomous clinical judgment: that they saw the patient completely, assessed the situation accurately, anticipated the risks, engaged the right colleagues, and acted within a specialty-informed, evidence-based framework.

That is nursopathic medicine in practice.

Clinical Reflection: Two Lenses, One Clinician

I hold two certifications: Family Nurse Practitioner and Psychiatric-Mental Health Nurse Practitioner. In practice, this means I carry two specialty lenses, and the experience of moving between them has taught me more about Specialty Lens Reasoning than any theoretical framework could.

My primary practice is psychiatric. When a patient presents for a mental health appointment, my PMHNP lens activates immediately and completely. Before the patient finishes their first sentence, I am observing their appearance, their psychomotor activity, the pace and pressure of their speech, whether their affect matches the content of what they are describing. When I open the Objective section of my SOAP note, I am writing a Mental Status Examination. I am not running through a physical systems review. The MSE is not supplemental to my assessment; it is my assessment. It is the observational instrument my training built.

But I practice in a telehealth setting where patients sometimes bring medical concerns to a psychiatric appointment. A patient managing anxiety or panic attacks may mention chest pain, a presentation where the somatic and psychiatric pictures are genuinely intertwined. A patient on antipsychotic medication may report new-onset fatigue and weight gain. A patient I have known for three years discloses that she has not seen a primary care provider in two years and wonders whether I can help.

In those moments, I am aware of something that I can now name precisely: I shift lenses. The PMHNP lens does not disappear; I am always tracking the psychiatric picture. But I consciously activate the FNP lens alongside it. The Objective section of that note looks different. I am asking about constitutional symptoms, reviewing systems, thinking about cardiovascular and metabolic risk in a way that is distinctly primary care in its orientation. My Assessment considers medical differentials that would not have been in the foreground of a purely psychiatric note.

This dual-lens experience reveals something important about the nature of Specialty Lens Reasoning: the lens is not a limitation. It is a trained perceptual clarity. When I practice as a PMHNP, I am not a less complete clinician than an FNP. I am a clinician whose observational apparatus is calibrated for the specific domain of mental health, with precision that a generalist lens cannot replicate. The MSE I write after 20 minutes with a patient contains clinical data that no laboratory value or vital sign would capture. That data is real, it is diagnostic, and it requires a specialty lens to gather.

What I have also learned is that holding two lenses does not mean applying both simultaneously to everything. Specialty Lens Reasoning requires knowing which lens is primary for this patient, in this encounter, for this purpose. The skill is not in having multiple lenses, but in knowing which one to look through, and when.

What I have come to understand about the five reasoning methods is that they are not a checklist or a sequence. They are a thought process: simultaneous, overlapping, and continuous from the moment a patient speaks their first word to the moment the encounter closes. Acute Reasoning is asking whether something is happening right now that requires immediate action. Longitudinal Reasoning is asking how this moment fits into everything I know about this patient across time. Anticipatory Reasoning is already looking ahead at what could go wrong if I don't act now. Interdisciplinary Reasoning is evaluating whether this exceeds what I can manage alone. And the Specialty Lens is filtering all of it through the clinical framework my training built. None of these pause while the others run. They run together.

The SOAP note is where that thought process gets transcribed. When I sit down to write after an encounter, I am not filling out a form. I am translating a cognitive event into a legible clinical record. The Subjective captures what the patient reported and what it signaled to me. The Objective captures what my lens trained me to look for and measure. The Assessment is where all five reasoning methods converge into a working diagnosis and differential. The Plan is where the reasoning becomes action. A rigorous SOAP note does not just document what happened. It makes the thinking visible to colleagues, to reviewers, and to the clinician themselves on the next visit when the trajectory needs to be understood. The reasoning methods are the thought. The SOAP note is the transcription of that thought. The chapters that follow on Acute Care, Chronic Care, Preventative Care, Interdisciplinary Care, and Specialty Care are where that transcription gets put into practice across the full range of clinical settings where NPs work.

Chapter 12 explores the formal boundaries of Specialty Lens Reasoning, including the certification requirements, scope alignment, and professional obligations that govern specialty practice in nursopathic medicine. The dual-lens experience described here is only possible because both lenses are grounded in formal graduate education and national certification. The lens is not something a clinician acquires by working in a setting. It is something they develop through training, validate through certification, and refine through sustained specialty practice.

CHAPTER SUMMARY

The five methods of clinical reasoning introduced in this chapter are the cognitive infrastructure of autonomous practice. They are not abstract principles; they are the actual mental operations that distinguish an expert clinician from a competent one.

The SOAP note is where these methods become visible. Every section of a rigorous note reflects simultaneous reasoning across multiple methods, with the Assessment as the primary site of convergence and the Plan as the expression of what that reasoning requires.

Specialty Lens Reasoning gives these differences their theoretical grounding. The PMHNP and the FNP do not simply reach different conclusions from the same observations. They make different observations, because they have been trained to notice different things. That is not a limitation of either clinician. It is what specialty preparation produces.

Together, they form the intellectual architecture of nursopathic medicine.

CHAPTER 4
PRACTICE QUESTIONS

MULTIPLE CHOICE QUESTIONS

1. **The five methods of clinical reasoning in nursopathic medicine correspond to:**
   A. The five steps of the nursing process
   B. The five practice domains of the nursopathic medicine model
   C. The five levels of Bloom's taxonomy
   D. The five stages of professional formation

2. **The core clinical question of Acute Reasoning is:**
   A. How has this patient changed over time?
   B. What harm can I anticipate and prevent?
   C. What is happening right now, and what must I do?
   D. How does my specialty shape what I observe?

3 **Longitudinal Reasoning differs from single-encounter reasoning primarily in that it:**
   A. Requires physician oversight across visits
   B. Holds diagnoses as evolving hypotheses refined across repeated encounters
   C. Only applies to primary care settings
   D. Eliminates the need for Acute Reasoning

4 Anticipatory Reasoning is best described as:

A. Reactive treatment of presenting symptoms

B. Protocol-driven screening checklists

C. Forward-looking clinical judgment that identifies and acts on foreseeable risks before they manifest

D. A reasoning method exclusive to preventive care visits

5. The distinction between Interdisciplinary Reasoning and dependency is:

A. Dependency is appropriate in states with restricted practice authority

B. Interdisciplinary Reasoning produces purposeful clinical collaboration; dependency produces deference regardless of clinical indication

C. Dependency is the same as referral

D. There is no meaningful clinical distinction

6. Specialty Lens Reasoning differs from the other four reasoning methods in that it:

A. Only applies to board-certified subspecialists

B. Operates across the entire SOAP note as a pervasive filter, rather than being localized to specific sections

C. Replaces the need for Acute and Longitudinal Reasoning

D. Is only relevant in tertiary care settings

7. A PMHNP and an FNP both see the same patient complaining of fatigue and insomnia. The fact that they generate different Objective sections primarily illustrates:

A. That one clinician is more thorough than the other

B. Specialty Lens Reasoning—each practitioner's training equips them with a different primary observational instrument

C. A disagreement about evidence-based practice

D. Scope of practice violation by one of the clinicians

8. In the SOAP note, the Assessment section simultaneously activates which reasoning methods?

A. Only Acute Reasoning

B. Only Longitudinal and Anticipatory Reasoning

C. Acute, Longitudinal, Anticipatory, and Interdisciplinary Reasoning—filtered by Specialty Lens Reasoning

D. Only the reasoning method most relevant to the chief complaint

9. An NP who recognizes that a patient's presenting complaint exceeds their scope and initiates a specialist referral is demonstrating:

A. A failure of autonomous practice

B. Interdisciplinary Reasoning—scope boundary recognition as an expression of professional responsibility

C. Dependency on physician oversight

D. A violation of the NP's practice authority

10. The SOAP note is described in this chapter as a "shared clinical language" because:

A. It is a standardized billing format used across specialties

B. It provides a common structure through which all five reasoning methods operate within a single clinical encounter

C. It is required by all state licensing boards

D. It replaces the need for documentation of clinical reasoning

CASE-BASED APPLICATION QUESTIONS

Case Scenario 1:

Alicia, a PMHNP, is seeing Marcus, a 38-year-old with bipolar II disorder, in a telehealth follow-up. He reports feeling "pretty good," sleeping 4 hours a night, and having started three new business projects in the past week. His mood is elevated but he denies feeling "manic." He was on lamotrigine 200 mg but stopped it two weeks ago because "I feel great and don't think I need it."

Questions:

- Identify which reasoning methods are active in this encounter and what each one is detecting.
- Walk through Alicia's SOAP note: What does Specialty Lens Reasoning shape in her Subjective section? What does Longitudinal Reasoning contribute to her Assessment?
- How does Acute Reasoning apply even though this is an outpatient telehealth follow-up?
- What Anticipatory Reasoning should Alicia document in her Plan?
- Is Interdisciplinary Reasoning indicated? If so, what type of interface and with whom?

Case Scenario 2:

James, an FNP, sees a new patient, Elena (age 51), for a wellness visit. She is a smoker (15 pack-years), works as a schoolteacher, has a family history of breast cancer (mother) and heart disease (father), and has been experiencing night sweats and irregular periods for eight months. Today her BP is 138/86, BMI is 28.5, and she mentions she has been "more anxious and forgetful" lately.

Questions:

- Map all five reasoning methods onto James's initial assessment of Elena. What is each method asking?

- James is an FNP. How does his Specialty Lens differ from how a PMHNP or a women's health NP might approach the same chief complaints?
- Write the Assessment section of James's SOAP note, demonstrating at least three reasoning methods explicitly.
- What Interdisciplinary Reasoning is required in this case, and which interface type (consultation, referral, co-management, or coordination) is appropriate for each?

TRUE/FALSE SELF-ASSESSMENT

1. ______ The five reasoning methods in nursopathic medicine operate sequentially, one at a time, within a clinical encounter.
2. ______ Specialty Lens Reasoning applies across all sections of the SOAP note, functioning as a pervasive filter.
3. ______ Acute Reasoning is defined by the setting (emergency department or hospital) rather than the cognitive operations involved.
4. ______ Longitudinal Reasoning holds every diagnosis as a working hypothesis subject to revision across repeated encounters.
5. ______ Anticipatory Reasoning applies only during wellness visits and primary care encounters.

See Appendix B for complete answers and rationales.

CHAPTER 5

EDUCATION AND PROFESSIONAL FORMATION IN NURSOPATHIC MEDICINE

LEARNING OBJECTIVES

Upon completing this chapter, students will be able to:

Explain how graduate nursing education functions as professional formation, meaning the structured development of clinical reasoning, ethical responsibility, and autonomous judgment, rather than simple skill acquisition.

Describe the cognitive shift from the RN role to the NP role and explain why this transition requires a fundamental reorientation of professional identity, not only additional knowledge or clinical experience.

Analyze how inadequate formation during the RN-to-NP transition can produce imposter syndrome, and explain how preceptorship, mentorship, and acceptance of clinical limits mitigate this experience.

Analyze how precepted clinical experience and mentorship develop the reasoning capacities required for autonomous practice, and how the specialty lens described in Chapter 4 is built through education and clinical formation rather than prior RN experience.

Evaluate the relationship between certification scope and employment setting, and apply this distinction to clinical scenarios involving scope boundary questions.

Articulate why lifelong learning is a professional obligation rather than a credential requirement, and how continuing education, reflective practice, and mentorship sustain autonomous competence over a career.

Apply the principle that independence is not conferred at graduation but developed through structured education, supervised clinical experience, and sustained professional responsibility.

Identify the ethical obligations that accompany autonomous practice authority, including recognition of limits and commitment to evidence-based standards, and explain how formation instills these obligations rather than merely teaching them.

CRITICAL THINKING QUESTIONS

Professional Formation: How does "professional formation" differ from traditional views of nursing education as skill-building? What are the implications for how NP programs should be designed and evaluated?

The RN-to-NP Transition: An experienced RN with fifteen years in critical care enters an AGACNP program. This clinician is technically skilled and knowledgeable, but the preceptor observes a consistent pattern of deferring clinical decisions upward rather than committing to an independent assessment and plan. What is happening, and what does NP education need to develop that years of RN experience did not?

Preceptorship: What distinguishes a formative preceptor relationship from one that merely logs clinical hours? What qualities would you look for in a preceptor, and what would you recognize as evidence that formation is actually occurring?

Scope Boundaries: A family NP is offered a position independently managing complex heart failure patients at a salary significantly higher than the current role. Using the principles from this chapter, what is the precise professional question that must be answered before accepting, and what does the responsible path forward look like?

RN Experience and the Specialty Lens: Many experienced clinicians argue that prior RN experience in a specialty area makes for a better NP in that specialty. Others argue that the NP role is a fundamentally different clinical role in which the lens matters more than the background setting, and that formation through graduate education builds the relevant capacity regardless of prior specialty experience. Which position do you find more persuasive, and why?

Evaluation: The chapter states that "independence is not conferred at graduation, but developed through structured education, supervised clinical experience, and sustained professional responsibility." What does this mean for new graduate NPs who are practicing with full authority on day one? Is there tension between regulatory autonomy and developmental readiness?

Synthesis: Design a clinical rotation or preceptorship that would specifically develop Longitudinal Reasoning, the capacity to hold a patient's trajectory in mind across time. What would that rotation look like, and how would you know whether it succeeded?

1. INTRODUCTION: EDUCATION AS FORMATION

Education is the primary mechanism through which autonomous practice is developed, sustained, and regulated within nursing. In nursopathic medicine, education is understood not merely as skill acquisition but as professional formation: the structured development of clinical reasoning, ethical responsibility, and accountability required for autonomous practice.

This distinction matters. Skill acquisition produces competence at defined tasks. Professional formation produces autonomous clinicians: practitioners who can hold an ambiguous clinical presentation in mind, generate a working hypothesis, reason through uncertainty, assume full responsibility for a decision, and revise that decision as new information arrives. Both the RN and the NP require deep clinical formation. What differs is the scope of the authority that formation is preparing them to carry.

This chapter addresses the architecture of that formation: the biomedical foundation that makes independent decision-making possible, the cognitive and identity shift required in the transition from RN to NP, the role of preceptorship and mentorship in building clinical reasoning, the scope boundaries that certification defines and employment cannot override, and the ongoing commitment to learning that sustains competence after the degree is conferred.

2. THE BIOMEDICAL FOUNDATION

Graduate nursing education has evolved to include advanced pathophysiology, pharmacology, health assessment, and specialty-specific clinical training. Within the nursopathic framework, these are not peripheral additions grafted onto a nursing curriculum. They are the cognitive substrate of autonomous practice, what makes independent diagnostic and therapeutic decision-making possible.

Advanced pathophysiology builds the conceptual model of the body that allows a clinician to reason from symptoms backward to cause and forward to consequence. Pharmacology provides the framework for understanding how interventions interact with pathophysiology: mechanism, kinetics, monitoring, and individualization. Health assessment, including both physical examination and the Mental Status Examination, is the primary data-gathering instrument of autonomous practice. These components, taken together, are what the NP draws on when authoring a clinical plan rather than carrying one out.

Within the nursopathic framework, biomedical knowledge is filtered through nursing's patient-centered orientation, ethical commitments, and attention to context and trajectory. The same pharmacology taught in a medical school is taught in NP programs—but applied through nursing's ways of knowing, which attend as much to the patient's experience of illness as to its biochemistry (Meleis, 2018).

3. THE RN-TO-NP COGNITIVE TRANSITION

Most nurse practitioners enter graduate education as registered nurses with clinical experience, sometimes years of it. This experience is genuinely valuable and not incidental. It builds pattern recognition, procedural fluency, clinical intuition, and a hard-won understanding of how patients move through the healthcare system. What RN experience does not automatically confer, however, is autonomous clinical authority. Recognizing that distinction is one of the most important transitions NP education facilitates.

The registered nurse role is a demanding clinical role in its own right. RNs assess patients continuously, recognize deterioration, advocate at the bedside, coordinate care across disciplines, and exercise real clinical judgment that directly affects patient outcomes. An experienced RN who holds a blood pressure medication on a hypotensive patient, or who escalates a subtle change in mental status before the rest of the team has noticed, is practicing with skill and clinical intelligence that should not be minimized. The RN's accountability is for the quality and safety of care delivery—and that accountability is significant.

What distinguishes the NP role is a different structure of authority, not a higher quality of care. The NP is the clinician who authors the diagnosis, the treatment plan, the prescriptions, the follow-up strategy, and the long-term clinical trajectory. Where the RN exercises clinical judgment within a framework of care that others have established, the NP is responsible for establishing that framework in the first place. The NP is, in the most direct sense, the captain of the patient's care—not because that role is more important than the RN's, but because it carries a different and complete set of clinical accountabilities. It is this difference in the structure of authority, not a difference in clinical worth, that NP education is designed to develop.

That shift in accountability requires a corresponding shift in cognitive orientation that RN experience, however extensive, does not automatically produce. The experienced RN entering an NP program often knows more clinical content than the program formally requires. What must be developed is not more information but a different relationship to clinical authority—the capacity to author the plan rather than execute it, to tolerate the weight of diagnostic uncertainty without deferring it to someone else, and be willing to say "this is my clinical judgment" and stand behind it (Benner, 1984).

4. IMPOSTER SYNDROME AND THE FORMATION GAP

When the transition from RN to NP is treated as content acquisition rather than identity formation, something predictable happens in the clinician who graduates: they step into autonomous practice carrying unresolved doubt about whether their authority is legitimate. They know the material. They passed the boards. But inside the clinical encounter, when a patient presents with an atypical picture, or a treatment decision requires standing behind a judgment without a physician to confirm it, a quiet but corrosive question surfaces: am I really qualified for this?

That experience has a name. Imposter syndrome—the persistent internalized belief that one's competence is insufficient despite objective evidence to the contrary—is widely documented among nurses and nursing students, with prevalence notably elevated during professional transitions into advanced and autonomous roles (Clance & Imes, 1978; Peng et al., 2022). It is not a personal failing. It is a predictable consequence of entering autonomous practice without adequate formation. When the educational process produces a clinician who has accumulated hours and passed examinations but has not been required to genuinely own clinical decisions during training, graduation creates a sudden and unbraced exposure to the full weight of autonomous accountability. The doubt that follows is rational. The formation gap is real.

I have experienced it myself, and I know many clinicians who have. What I have learned, and what those clinicians consistently report, is that the resolution does not come from knowing more. It comes from acceptance: accepting what you know and accepting what you do not know with equal honesty. New NPs often emerge from training believing they must know everything. The expectation is comprehensive mastery. And when the first genuinely uncertain clinical moment arrives, and it always does, the gap between that expectation and the reality of clinical uncertainty can feel like evidence of inadequacy. It is not. It is evidence of practicing at the frontier of actual clinical complexity, which is exactly where autonomous practice lives.

What mitigates imposter syndrome is not the elimination of uncertainty but the development of a healthy relationship with it. That relationship is built through two mechanisms. The first is adequate formation during training: preceptored experience in which the student is required to reason independently, hold clinical uncertainty without immediate resolution, and take accountability for decisions before the preceptor intervenes. A student who has been through that process knows, by the time of graduation, that uncertainty is manageable. They have evidence, from their own clinical experience, that they can think through what they do not know and arrive at a defensible judgment. The second mechanism is mentorship after graduation: access to experienced clinicians who normalize uncertainty, model how seasoned practitioners handle the limits of their own knowledge, and provide a safe structure within which the new NP can continue to develop without the amplifying isolation of practicing alone.

Knowing your limitations is not a deficit. It is a clinical skill. The NP who accurately recognizes when a presentation exceeds their current expertise and initiates a referral or consultation is not demonstrating inadequacy; they are demonstrating exactly the kind of autonomous clinical judgment that formation is designed to produce. This is where interdisciplinary care enters not as a concession but as a strength. Referral and consultation are not evidence that the NP is less than. They are evidence that the NP understands something sophisticated: that together, across disciplines, patient care improves in ways that no single clinician, regardless of credential, can replicate alone. The NP who refers appropriately is not practicing beneath their scope. They are practicing at its best expression.

The formation process described in this chapter (graduate education, preceptored clinical experience, and sustained mentorship) is the infrastructure that makes this acceptance possible. It does not eliminate imposter syndrome by producing omniscience. It eliminates it by producing clinicians who are grounded enough in their own formation to know what they know, honest enough to know what they do not, and confident enough in both to practice with integrity.

5. PRECEPTORSHIP, MENTORSHIP, AND THE SPECIALTY LENS

Precepted clinical experience is the site where professional formation actually happens. This is not a regulatory formality. It is the educational mechanism through which clinical reasoning is built, tested, and refined in real conditions with real patients. Hours alone do not accomplish this. What matters is the cognitive work that occurs within those hours: whether the student generates the differential before the preceptor offers it, whether the student defends the assessment and revises it when challenged, whether genuine clinical uncertainty is experienced and met with action rather than avoidance.

The preceptor relationship is the most influential educational relationship in NP formation. A skilled preceptor does not demonstrate correct answers. A skilled preceptor creates conditions in which the student must reason—requiring written differentials before discussion, asking the student to present before examining, allowing decisions to stand and then reviewing their consequences. This kind of preceptorship builds the clinical mind rather than filling it (Tanner, 2006).

A question frequently raised among colleagues in NP education is whether prior RN experience in a specialty (inpatient psychiatry, critical care, emergency medicine) makes for a better NP in that specialty. Many experienced practitioners argue that it does, and the argument is not without merit. Task familiarity, environment knowledge, and comfort with the patient population can ease the clinical transition. But the NP role is a fundamentally different role in which the lens matters more than the background setting. As Chapter 4 establishes, the specialty lens is a cognitive framework—a pervasive filter through which training, certification, and population focus shape every clinical observation and every decision. That lens is built through graduate education and sustained clinical immersion, not through prior RN experience in the setting.

A clinician who completed an FNP program and subsequently developed a psychiatric mental health practice has developed a specialty lens through the work of that practice, through the accumulation of clinical encounters, through reflection and mentorship, through the sustained application of psychiatric diagnostic reasoning to a defined population. The lens is different from what a PMHNP's training specifically develops, but it is a functional clinical lens nonetheless. The NP role remains the same across both certifications: the clinician leads patient care, authors the plan, and holds full clinical accountability. What changes is the lens through which that practice is conducted—not the fundamental structure of the role.

Mentorship extends this formative work beyond graduation. The new graduate NP benefits from access to experienced practitioners who can review complex cases, discuss clinical uncertainty, and model the kind of sustained professional judgment that a two-year program can only begin to develop. Formal mentorship programs, peer consultation structures, and ongoing professional community engagement are continuations of the formative process that graduation interrupts but does not complete (Hamric et al., 2014).

6. ETHICAL FORMATION AND AUTONOMOUS ACCOUNTABILITY

Ethical formation is woven through every clinical encounter in which a student must decide what responsible autonomous practice looks like when the answer is not obvious. Nursing ethics, grounded in beneficence, patient advocacy, and relational responsibility,provides the moral framework within which autonomous clinical decisions are made (Beauchamp & Childress, 2019; Grace, 2018). This framework shapes practice in ways a purely biomedical model does not.

Autonomous practice amplifies these ethical obligations because it removes the diffusion of responsibility that comes from shared clinical authority. When the NP is the clinician accountable for a decision, the ethical weight of that decision rests entirely with that clinician. Formation builds the capacity to carry that weight—including the recognition that knowing when a presentation exceeds one's expertise and initiating appropriate consultation is not a failure of autonomy but one of its most important expressions (Hamric et al., 2014).

7. SCOPE, CERTIFICATION, AND THE EMPLOYMENT TRAP

One of the most consequential misunderstandings in NP practice is the belief that employment in a specialty setting confers specialty scope. It does not. Scope of practice is determined by graduate education and national certification, not by the clinical environment, not by institutional credentialing, and not by years of on-the-job exposure in a specialty area (NCSBN, 2008).

An FNP employed in a cardiology specialty clinic practices within FNP scope regardless of the clinical sophistication of the role. An AGPCNP hired to cover a pediatric unit does not acquire pediatric scope through exposure. The professional and legal consequences of practicing outside certification scope fall entirely on the clinician, not the institution. The responsible path when scope and clinical role are misaligned is to obtain appropriate preparation—additional training, subspecialty certification where available, and honest self-assessment about what currently falls within one's clinical competency.

The principle is consistent throughout nursopathic medicine: authority must be matched with competency, and competency in a specialty is built through education, not exposure.

8. LIFELONG LEARNING AS PROFESSIONAL OBLIGATION

Autonomous practice is not a destination. Clinical evidence evolves, guidelines are revised, new treatments emerge, and patient populations change. The clinician who exits a graduate program with credentials for autonomous practice has completed a formation process—but formation does not end at graduation.

Continuing education, certification maintenance, and reflective practice are therefore not bureaucratic requirements. They are the ongoing mechanisms of professional formation. The clinician who treats them as boxes to check has misunderstood the nature of the obligation. Lifelong learning is what sustains the alignment between the authority autonomous practice confers and the competency that authority demands (Melnyk & Fineout-Overholt, 2019; DiCenso et al., 2005).

Reflective practice is particularly important. The formed clinician develops the habit of reviewing clinical decisions routinely, not only after adverse outcomes. What did I miss? Was my differential complete? Did I act too quickly or too slowly? Did my specialty lens reveal something important, or did it narrow my view? This kind of ongoing self-audit is what separates autonomous practice from the assumption of competence.

9. CONCLUSION: STRUCTURED DEVELOPMENT

By framing education as professional formation, nursopathic medicine offers a coherent explanation for how nurse practitioners are prepared for autonomous practice. Independence is not conferred at graduation. It is developed through structured education, supervised clinical experience, and sustained professional responsibility, maintained through a career defined by lifelong learning and reflective practice.

The specialty lens and the reasoning methods described in Chapter 4 are not separate from this formation. They are its content and its product. The NP who has undergone genuine professional formation does not practice differently because of additional credentials. The difference is in having developed a specific structure of clinical authority—one that carries full accountability for the diagnosis, the plan, and the outcome from the first encounter to the last.

Clinical Reflection: "I'm Going to Make You a Great Clinician"

The debate about whether prior RN experience makes a better NP is one I have heard throughout my career, and I have a personal stake in it. My colleagues who completed inpatient psychiatric rotations as RNs before entering PMHNP programs sometimes suggest that not having that background puts a clinician at a disadvantage. I never worked in an inpatient crisis unit as an RN. I did not have psychiatric RN experience before I entered NP training. What I did have was several years of FNP practice, a specialty lens built through direct patient care, and a preceptor who shaped the way I practice to this day.

He was a DO running his own private family medicine practice, the kind of physician who treated patients as people rather than diagnoses. He had been in practice for decades and had a reputation among his patients that was built less on credentials than on the quality of attention he gave in the room. Before one of our early clinical sessions, he told me something I have never forgotten: "I'm going to make you a great clinician that stands out." I did not fully understand what he meant at the time. I was focused on learning clinical content. He was trying to teach me something different.

What he was teaching was not primarily biomedical knowledge, though he taught that too. It was the kind of clinician he believed the role demanded. He actively listened to patients, not the polite half-attention that passes for listening in busy clinical settings, but genuine, present attention that allowed him to understand not just what was wrong but who was sitting in front of him. He took care to get to know his patients on a personal level, building relationships that made clinical trust possible. He used to say: "It's not how much you know, but how much you care." That principle has stayed with me, and it is something I practice at my own telehealth practice today.

He also taught me specific clinical reasoning. He was the one who first explained C-peptide testing to me, walking me through the logic of using it to distinguish late-onset type 1 from type 2 diabetes—what the test measures, why it matters, when to order it. Who would have thought that I would not only be applying that teaching in my first NP job, diagnosing a patient with LADA and initiating insulin while the medical director argued for metformin, but that I would still be talking about it more than a decade later in this book? That is what a formative preceptor does. He does not just show you a clinical answer. He builds the reasoning that makes you reach for the right question.

My FNP experience has proven more directly useful in my psychiatric practice than any inpatient psychiatric RN experience might have been. The FNP lens trained me to think medically, to hold the whole patient, to consider physical illness as a contributor to psychiatric presentation, to recognize when a depressed patient's fatigue needs a metabolic workup rather than an antidepressant adjustment. As Chapter 4 describes, the specialty lens changes the clinical filter through which you see a patient, but the NP role itself remains constant: you are leading care, authoring the plan, holding full accountability for what happens next. My lens shifted when I moved from family medicine to psychiatric practice. My role did not.

The colleague who worries that I lack something by not having inpatient psychiatric RN experience may be right that there are things I would have learned in that setting. But formation does not come from exposure alone. It comes from the quality of clinical experience, from preceptors who hold you to the standard of reasoning rather than the standard of task completion, and from the accumulation of clinical encounters through which a specialty lens is genuinely built. My preceptor's voice—"it's not how much you know, but how much you care"—is not a soft sentiment. It is a clinical epistemology. And it is one that nursopathic medicine, grounded in nursing's relational tradition and its commitment to the whole patient, has always understood.

CHAPTER SUMMARY

Education in nursopathic medicine is professional formation: the structured development of clinical reasoning, ethical responsibility, and autonomous accountability required for independent practice. The RN-to-NP transition requires not just additional knowledge but a fundamental reorientation of professional identity—from a role defined by clinical excellence within an established framework of care to a role defined by establishing that framework directly and holding complete accountability for the clinical decisions it contains. Both roles demand genuine clinical competence. What the NP role adds is a different and complete structure of clinical authority.

Precepted clinical experience and mentorship are the primary mechanisms through which professional formation happens. The specialty lens described in Chapter 4 is built through graduate education and sustained clinical immersion rather than through prior RN experience in a specialty setting. Prior RN experience offers genuine value, but the NP role is a different role, and the lens required for that role is built through formation, not background. Scope of practice is determined by certification, not employment. Lifelong learning, reflective practice, and ongoing mentorship sustain the alignment between autonomous authority and the competency it demands throughout a career.

CHAPTER 5
PRACTICE QUESTIONS

Multiple Choice Questions

1. **Education in nursopathic medicine is understood primarily as:**
   A. Skill acquisition and task training
   B. Professional formation: the structured development of clinical reasoning, ethical responsibility, and autonomous accountability
   C. Preparation for certification examinations
   D. Apprenticeship in physician-led clinical practice

2. **The primary difference between the RN role and the NP role is:**
   A. The NP has more clinical experience and knowledge
   B. The NP leads patient care directly, authoring the diagnosis and treatment plan and holding full clinical accountability for the outcome
   C. The NP works without physician oversight
   D. The NP has completed more years of total clinical training

3. **An experienced RN entering an NP program most needs to develop:**
   A. More biomedical knowledge than the program formally requires
   B. A different relationship to clinical authority—the capacity to author clinical decisions independently and hold full accountability for their outcomes
   C. Faster clinical decision-making skills
   D. Comfort with physician supervision

4. What distinguishes preceptored clinical experience that builds autonomous reasoning from experience that merely fulfills hour requirements?

A. The total number of clinical hours completed

B. The student observing experienced clinicians manage complex cases

C. The student being required to reason independently, defend clinical judgments, and take accountability for decisions before the preceptor intervenes

D. Rotating through the greatest variety of clinical settings

5. Scope of practice for a nurse practitioner is determined by:

A. The specialty of the clinical setting in which they are employed

B. Years of clinical experience in a specialty area

C. Graduate education and national certification

D. Institutional credentialing and hospital privileges

6. A preceptor who is doing genuine formative work will:

A. Demonstrate correct clinical answers for the student to observe

B. Ensure the student completes the required number of clinical hours efficiently

C. Create conditions in which the student must reason independently, defend judgments, and take responsibility for clinical decisions

D. Provide close supervision for every patient encounter

7. **Ethical formation in nursopathic medicine includes:**
   A. Memorizing nursing ethics codes
   B. Developing recognition of limits, appropriate consultation, and commitment to evidence-based standards as intrinsic professional obligations
   C. Deferring ethically complex decisions to physicians
   D. Following institutional protocols without deviation

8. **An FNP who accepts a position independently managing complex heart failure patients without appropriate preparation is:**
   A. Expanding scope appropriately through specialty employment
   B. Practicing outside certification scope regardless of institutional support for the role
   C. Demonstrating advanced professional formation
   D. Exercising the interdisciplinary care domain

9. **Lifelong learning in autonomous practice is best understood as:**
   A. A regulatory requirement to maintain licensure
   B. A professional obligation that sustains the alignment between autonomous authority and the competency that authority demands
   C. Optional for NPs with more than ten years of experience
   D. Equivalent to attending annual conferences

10. **Independence in nurse practitioner practice is:**
    A. Conferred automatically at graduation and certification
    B. Developed through structured education, supervised clinical experience, and sustained professional responsibility—and maintained through lifelong learning
    C. Granted by the employing institution
    D. Not achievable without physician collaboration

CASE-BASED APPLICATION QUESTIONS

Case Scenario 1:

Jennifer just graduated from an FNP program and is offered a position in a busy orthopedic surgery practice managing pre- and post-operative patients. The salary is excellent, but the role involves managing complex orthopedic conditions and post-surgical complications not covered in the FNP training. The orthopedic surgeon says Jennifer will "pick it up quickly" on the job.

Questions:

- What is the precise scope question Jennifer must answer before accepting this position, and why does the surgeon's confidence in Jennifer's learning capacity not resolve it?
- How does employment setting relate to, and specifically not expand, certification scope?
- What would a responsible path forward look like if Jennifer genuinely wants to practice in orthopedic surgery?

Case Scenario 2:

Marcus is an experienced PMHNP who has been practicing for five years. He believes his experience is sufficient and sees no need for continuing education beyond the minimum required for license renewal. He states: "I learned everything I need in graduate school and from experience."

Questions:

- How does Marcus's attitude conflict with the concept of professional formation as lifelong rather than terminal?
- Why is experience alone insufficient to sustain autonomous competence, and what specifically does continuing education address that experience cannot?
- What are the ethical implications of this approach for Marcus's patients?

TRUE/FALSE SELF-ASSESSMENT

1. ______ Education in nursopathic medicine is primarily about acquiring clinical skills and biomedical knowledge.
2. ______ The RN-to-NP transition is primarily a matter of learning new content rather than a reorientation of professional identity and clinical authority.
3. ______ Employment in a specialty clinic automatically expands a nurse practitioner's scope of practice.
4. ______ Scope of practice is determined by graduate education and national certification, not by employment setting.
5. ______ Lifelong learning is a professional obligation that sustains autonomous competence, not merely a regulatory requirement.

See Appendix B for complete answers and rationales.

CHAPTER 6

REGULATORY IMPLICATIONS OF NURSOPATHIC MEDICINE

LEARNING OBJECTIVES

Upon completing this chapter, students will be able to:

Describe how current regulatory models define NP scope through licensure, certification, and statutory authority.

Compare independent, reduced, and restricted practice authority models in the U.S.

Explain how nursopathic medicine provides conceptual clarity without requiring statutory changes.

Analyze regulatory variability across U.S. states and international jurisdictions.

Identify similarities and differences in advanced practice regulation across multiple countries (Canada, UK, Australia, New Zealand, etc.).

Evaluate how the five-domain model applies across diverse international regulatory frameworks.

Apply principles from international models to inform U.S. regulatory discussions.

CRITICAL THINKING QUESTIONS

Comparative Analysis: Using Appendix A, compare advanced practice regulation in three different countries. What common challenges do they face? How do their solutions differ?

Application: You're advocating for full practice authority in your state. How would you use the nursopathic medicine framework (rather than just outcome data or workforce arguments) to support your position?

International Perspective: The chapter describes how Canada's provincial variation creates a "natural experiment" in regulatory approaches. What can the U.S. learn from provinces with full autonomy versus those with restrictions?

Role Clarity: How does providing a clear theoretical framework for NP practice potentially reduce regulatory confusion even without changing laws? Give specific examples.

Evaluation: The chapter states that nursopathic medicine "affirms current regulatory structures while providing nursing with a coherent explanation." Is this a strength or weakness? Should the framework push for regulatory change rather than accepting current structures?

Synthesis: If you were designing advanced practice regulation for a country just establishing NP roles, what key principles from this chapter would guide your approach? Why?

Critical Thinking: Some jurisdictions require "collaborative agreements" that may be difficult to obtain, creating de facto barriers to practice. How does nursopathic medicine's emphasis on Interdisciplinary Care as a domain (rather than a regulatory requirement) address this issue?

1. INTRODUCTION: REGULATION AND CONCEPTUAL CLARITY

Regulation plays a central role in shaping autonomous practice, yet regulatory frameworks often describe what nurse practitioners may do without explaining how their authority functions within nursing. Nursopathic medicine does not seek to alter existing regulatory structures, but to provide conceptual clarity that supports consistent interpretation and implementation.

2. CURRENT REGULATORY MODELS

Current regulatory models define nurse practitioner scope through licensure, certification, and statutory authority. These mechanisms establish boundaries of practice, delineate accountability, and protect the public. Within this context, autonomous practice is recognized as a function of regulation rather than delegation. Nursopathic medicine aligns with this recognition by framing medical diagnosis and treatment as inherent components of advanced nursing practice within established scope.

3. ADDRESSING VARIABILITY

One regulatory challenge has been the variability in how autonomy is described across jurisdictions. Differences in language and structure can create confusion regarding professional roles and responsibilities. By offering a nursing-centered explanation of autonomous practice, nursopathic medicine supports clearer communication among regulators, educators, employers, and the public without requiring uniform statutory language.

4. PATIENT SAFETY AND ACCOUNTABILITY

Nursopathic medicine also reinforces regulatory priorities related to patient safety and accountability. By emphasizing evidence-based practice, ethical responsibility, and longitudinal management, the model aligns with regulatory expectations for competence and quality of care. Autonomy within this framework is accompanied by clear professional responsibility, mitigating concerns that independence equates to unregulated practice.

5. COLLABORATION AS CLINICAL NECESSITY

Interdisciplinary collaboration remains a regulatory consideration. Nursopathic medicine affirms collaboration as a clinical necessity rather than a regulatory constraint. Nurse practitioners practicing autonomously are expected to engage other professionals when clinically appropriate, consistent with standards of care and institutional policies. This expectation supports regulatory goals while preserving independent authority.

6. NOT SEEKING STATUTORY CHANGE

Importantly, nursopathic medicine does not propose new titles, licensure categories, or scope expansions. Its regulatory implication is conceptual rather than statutory: it offers a language through which existing autonomy can be understood, taught, and evaluated. By clarifying the nature of autonomous practice, the model may reduce ambiguity and support more consistent regulatory interpretation over time.

7. INTERNATIONAL PERSPECTIVES ON ADVANCED PRACTICE REGULATION

While this text has focused primarily on nurse practitioner practice in the United States, advanced practice nursing exists globally under various titles, regulatory frameworks, and scopes of practice. Examining international contexts demonstrates both the universality of the conceptual challenges nursopathic medicine addresses and the diversity of regulatory solutions that different healthcare systems have developed.

8. GLOBAL TERMINOLOGY AND ROLE VARIATION

Advanced practice nursing roles exist internationally under different names and organizational structures:

- **Advanced Nurse Practitioners** (**ANPs**) in the United Kingdom, Ireland, and many Commonwealth countries practice with varying degrees of autonomy depending on jurisdiction and setting (Bryant-Lukosius & DiCenso, 2004; Kleinpell et al., 2014).
- **Nurse Practitioners** in Canada operate under provincial/territorial regulation, with scope and autonomy varying significantly across the country. Some provinces grant full practice authority while others maintain collaborative practice requirements.

- **Nurse Practitioners** in Australia and New Zealand hold prescribing authority and practice with substantial autonomy, particularly in rural and underserved areas where access to physicians is limited.
- **Physician Assistants with Nursing Background** or specialized advanced nursing roles exist in the Netherlands, where "Nurse Specialists" practice autonomously within defined specialty areas.
- **Clinical Nurse Specialists** in many European countries perform advanced assessment and management functions that more closely resemble nurse practitioner practice than the traditional U.S. CNS consultation and education model, though regulatory frameworks vary widely across the European Union.

Despite different titles and regulatory structures, these international roles share common features when they engage in autonomous diagnostic and therapeutic practice: graduate-level education, advanced clinical decision-making authority, diagnostic and prescriptive functions, and responsibility for patient outcomes. Where international advanced practice roles operate within this diagnostic-therapeutic model. Regardless of what they are called, the five domains of nursopathic medicine. Acute Care, Chronic Care, Preventative Care, Interdisciplinary Care, and Specialty Care, apply, even when specific regulatory language differs.

9. COMPARATIVE REGULATORY MODELS

International advanced practice regulation reveals diverse approaches to structuring autonomy:

- **Full Practice Authority Models:** Countries like New Zealand grant nurse practitioners independent practice rights comparable to U.S. states with full practice authority (Delamaire & Lafortune, 2010). Nurse practitioners assess, diagnose, prescribe, and manage patients autonomously within their scope of practice.

- **Collaborative Practice Models:** The United Kingdom's system requires ANPs to work within agreed protocols and clinical governance frameworks, though the degree of physician involvement varies by NHS trust and specialty. This resembles U.S. reduced or restricted practice environments.
- **Hybrid Models:** Canada's provincial variation creates a natural experiment in regulatory approaches. Provinces like Alberta and Saskatchewan grant broader autonomy, while others maintain more restrictive frameworks. This variation within a single national healthcare system parallels U.S. state-by-state differences.
- **Emerging Models:** Countries like Ireland and several Scandinavian nations are actively developing and expanding advanced practice nursing roles, often learning from established models in North America and Oceania.

10. UNIVERSAL CHALLENGES AND THE NURSOPATHIC FRAMEWORK

Despite regulatory diversity, international advanced practice nursing faces similar conceptual challenges:

- **Role Clarity:** In many countries, the relationship between advanced practice nursing and medical practice remains under-theorized. Questions about whether ANPs/NPs "practice medicine" or "extend nursing" persist globally, mirroring the conceptual ambiguity this text addresses for U.S. nurse practitioners.
- **Scope Definition:** International debates about what activities fall within advanced nursing scope versus medical scope parallel U.S. discussions. The nursopathic framework's functional domain approach offers a language that transcends jurisdiction-specific statutory definitions.
- **Interprofessional Relationships:** Globally, advanced practice nurses navigate relationships with physicians, pharmacists, and other healthcare professionals. The Interdisciplinary Care

domain's emphasis on collaboration without subordination addresses a universal challenge.

- **Educational Preparation:** Most countries require master's-level education for advanced practice roles, recognizing that autonomous clinical authority demands graduate preparation (Kleinpell et al., 2014). This aligns with nursopathic medicine's emphasis on professional formation.
- **Evidence-Based Practice:** Regardless of country, advanced practice nursing is expected to operate within evidence-based standards. The foundational role of evidence-based practice in the nursopathic model applies universally.

11. APPLICABILITY OF THE FIVE-DOMAIN MODEL INTERNATIONALLY

The nursopathic medicine framework's functional organization makes it adaptable to diverse international contexts:

- **Acute Care** functions similarly across countries—ANPs/NPs manage urgent presentations, make timely diagnostic and therapeutic decisions, and assume responsibility for outcomes under time constraints.
- **Chronic Care** reflects the global shift toward managing aging populations and chronic disease. Advanced practice nurses worldwide provide longitudinal management, whether in the NHS, Canadian provincial health systems, or Australian practices.
- **Preventative Care** aligns with international health priorities around screening, immunization, and risk reduction, practiced within public health systems or private clinics depending on the country's healthcare structure.
- **Interdisciplinary Care** operates across all systems, though the specific professions and relationships vary. The core principle (autonomous authority within collaborative systems) remains constant.

- **Specialty Care** exists internationally through population-focused (pediatric, geriatric) or setting-focused (critical care, emergency) advanced practice roles, organized similarly to U.S. specialty NP practice.

The model's foundation in **Evidence-Based Practice** transcends national boundaries, as scientific evidence and clinical guidelines increasingly reflect international research and consensus..

12. REGULATORY DIVERSITY AND THEORETICAL UNITY

The international landscape reveals a striking pattern: while regulatory approaches vary significantly across jurisdictions, the functional nature of advanced practice nursing is broadly consistent. Nurse practitioners and advanced nursing practitioners worldwide exercise autonomous or semi-autonomous clinical judgment, integrate biomedical knowledge with nursing values, assume accountability for patient outcomes, and navigate interdisciplinary structures while maintaining professional identity. These functional commonalities persist regardless of whether practice occurs under a nationally unified regulatory framework or a fragmented provincial one—suggesting that nursopathic medicine, though developed from U.S. experience, articulates something universal about advanced nursing practice rather than something jurisdiction-specific.

Cross-national experience offers instructive reference points. Australia and Canada demonstrate that autonomous advanced practice can be structurally essential—not merely supplementary—in addressing geographic healthcare access disparities. The UK's integration of advanced nurse practitioners within the NHS shows how autonomous nursing roles function within centralized, publicly funded systems, distinct from the U.S. mixed public-private model. Countries with recently established advanced practice frameworks, including Ireland and several EU nations, demonstrate that coherent regulatory structures can be built relatively quickly when political will and professional consensus converge.

At the same time, the U.S. contributes its own export: the conceptual clarity that frameworks like nursopathic medicine offer for explaining autonomous practice as an extension of nursing identity rather than a departure from it. Internationally, that explanatory clarity is increasingly sought. Growing scholarship on advanced practice theory across multiple health systems reflects a shared need for frameworks that explain what advanced practice nurses do, not merely describe the tasks they perform or the titles they hold.

13. CONCLUSION: REGULATORY CLARITY AS PROFESSIONAL FOUNDATION

The international variation in regulatory structures underscores a point that is equally relevant domestically: regulatory frameworks define the legal parameters of practice, but they do not explain it. Whether a nurse practitioner operates under full practice authority in Arizona or within a collaborative framework in Alberta, the same clinical functions are being performed, the same professional accountability is engaged, and the same nursing identity is operative. What differs is the statutory architecture surrounding that practice—not the practice itself.

Nursopathic medicine addresses this gap. By providing a framework grounded in education, ethics, and evidence-based accountability rather than in any particular regulatory structure, it offers language that travels across jurisdictions. The five domains function regardless of state or national context. The model's emphasis on professional identity, autonomous authority, and accountability is as relevant to a nurse practitioner navigating an NHS trust as to one managing an independent panel in a full-practice state. Regulators, educators, and practitioners alike benefit when professional theory aligns with clinical reality—and that alignment, more than any single statutory change, is what this framework is designed to provide.

Clinical Reflection: Direct Primary Care and Insurance Barriers

I started my own practice in June 2020, in the middle of the COVID-19 pandemic—a time that made launching any healthcare business particularly challenging. I initially established a Direct Primary Care (DPC) model, which charges patients a monthly membership fee for primary care services rather than billing through insurance.

I chose DPC for several reasons that will be familiar to many nurse practitioners. The model enables direct relationships with patients, offers flexibility in visit length and care delivery, and aligns well with nursing's emphasis on holistic, patient-centered care. For me, an additional practical factor was relevant: nurse practitioners in some states and practice contexts encounter credentialing challenges with certain payers, which can create friction between state-granted practice authority and insurance participation. The DPC structure sidesteps this friction by design, making it a pragmatic option for clinicians navigating those gaps—whether they are drawn to it primarily for its care philosophy or its operational simplicity.

The DPC model has found success particularly in rural and underserved areas where accessible primary care is scarce. In metropolitan and suburban contexts, it tends to function more like concierge medicine, with patients paying out-of-pocket despite carrying insurance. I was in that latter situation—practicing in a suburban area where patients had insurance coverage and were generally disinclined to pay separately for primary care. I attracted only a small panel under that model. But the experience was formative. I learned to contain overhead, operate efficiently, and most importantly understanding what drives patient retention when the relationship is entirely voluntary: the value and quality of the care itself.

Eventually, I transitioned my practice to psychiatric mental health, drawing on my PMHNP certification. Several patients who had initially come to me for primary care followed me into that specialty, continuing under my care as I shifted focus. That continuity shaped the quality of the psychiatric care I could provide. I knew their histories, understood their contexts, had already built therapeutic trust. The transition from primary to psychiatric care wasn't a break in the relationship—it was an extension of it.

This experience illustrates something central to nursopathic medicine: nurse practitioners build sustained relationships over time, adapting clinical focus while maintaining the continuity that defines high-quality longitudinal care. The patients who moved with me weren't accessing a new service—they were continuing a relationship with a clinician who knew them whole. That longitudinal knowing is not incidental to psychiatric care. It is constitutive of it.

CHAPTER SUMMARY

Regulation defines the legal boundaries of nurse practitioner practice, but often lacks theoretical explanation of how autonomous authority functions. Nursopathic medicine provides conceptual clarity that supports consistent regulatory interpretation, reinforces patient safety priorities, and affirms collaboration without requiring statutory changes. The framework stabilizes autonomous practice by aligning theory with existing regulatory structures.

CHAPTER 6
PRACTICE QUESTIONS

MULTIPLE CHOICE QUESTIONS

1. **Current regulatory models define NP scope through:**
   A. Employment contracts
   B. Licensure, certification, and statutory authority
   C. Physician preference
   D. Hospital policies

2. **Nursopathic medicine's purpose regarding regulation is to:**
   A. Advocate for changing all state laws
   B. Provide conceptual clarity without requiring statutory changes
   C. Eliminate licensing requirements
   D. Create new regulatory categories

3. **Independent practice authority means:**
   A. NPs never collaborate with anyone
   B. Authority aligned with licensure and scope, with direct accountability
   C. No regulations apply
   D. Freedom to practice beyond scope

4. **Restrictive practice environments typically require:**
   A. Graduate education
   B. Mandated supervisory or collaborative arrangements
   C. National certification
   D. Continuing education

5. **Nursopathic medicine frames collaboration as:**
   A. A regulatory requirement
   B. A clinical necessity, not a regulatory constraint
   C. Unnecessary for NPs
   D. A sign of incompetence

6. **The chapter's regulatory implication is primarily:**
   A. Statutory
   B. Conceptual
   C. Financial
   D. International

7. **In Canada, advanced practice regulation:**
   A. Is uniform across all provinces
   B. Varies by province, similar to U.S. state variation
   C. Doesn't exist
   D. Is more restrictive than the U.S.

8. **The chapter emphasizes that nursopathic medicine does NOT propose:**
   A. A theoretical framework
   B. New titles, licensure categories, or scope expansions
   C. Evidence-based practice
   D. Professional accountability

9. **The five-domain model applies internationally because:**
   A. All countries have identical regulations
   B. It describes functional competencies rather than jurisdiction-specific tasks
   C. Only the U.S. has NPs
   D. International NPs are less qualified

10. Nursopathic medicine may reduce regulatory ambiguity by:

A. Changing all state laws

B. Offering a language for consistent interpretation without requiring uniform statutes

C. Eliminating regulations

D. Creating federal mandates

CASE-BASED APPLICATION QUESTIONS

Case Scenario 1:

State Representative Johnson is drafting legislation about NP practice. She has outcome data showing safety and effectiveness but remains confused about "what exactly is the NP role and how is it different from medicine?" She's considering requiring physician supervision "just to be safe."

Questions:

- How does nursopathic medicine provide conceptual clarity that outcome data alone cannot?
- Why might a theoretical framework reduce Representative Johnson's concerns more effectively than empirical data?
- How would you explain that collaboration ≠ supervision using the nursopathic framework?

Case Scenario 2:

Maria practices as an FNP in Alberta, Canada, which has relatively independent practice authority. She's considering relocating to a province with more restrictive regulations requiring collaborative agreements. She's concerned about maintaining autonomous practice.

Questions:

- How does regulatory structure affect practice differently than professional competence?

- Using Chapter 6's framework, how might Maria maintain professional autonomy even in restrictive environments?
- What does the chapter suggest about the relationship between regulation and professional identity?

TRUE/FALSE SELF-ASSESSMENT

1. ______ Nursopathic medicine advocates for immediate changes to all state practice acts.
2. ______ Independent practice authority means NPs practice without any professional accountability.
3. ______ Collaboration in nursopathic medicine is a clinical necessity, not a regulatory constraint.
4. ______ Canada's provincial variation in NP regulation parallels U.S. state variation.
5. ______ The five-domain model requires uniform statutory language to function.

See Appendix B for complete answers and rationales.

PART II

THE NURSOPATHIC MEDICINE PRACTICE MODEL

CHAPTER 7

THE NURSOPATHIC MEDICINE PRACTICE MODEL

LEARNING OBJECTIVES

Upon completing this chapter, students will be able to:

Describe the five domains of nursopathic medicine and explain how each functions across specialties.

Interpret the visual architectural model, including the symbolism of white marble, the green vine, and gold inscriptions.

Explain what the green vine on Interdisciplinary Care symbolizes and why balance matters (too tight constricts, too loose fumbles).

Analyze how evidence-based practice serves as the foundation for all five domains.

Apply the five-domain model to diverse specialty settings (psychiatric, acute care, primary care, etc.).

Evaluate how the model maintains coherence across different NP specialties while accommodating diversity.

Synthesize understanding of how all five domains integrate to constitute nursopathic medicine.

CRITICAL THINKING QUESTIONS

Visual Interpretation: Explain how the architectural metaphor (Roman columns, marble, vine, gold) conveys meaning beyond mere decoration. What would be lost if the model were just a simple list?

The Vine's Lesson: The green vine represents collaboration that is "balanced to neither constrict care nor fumble it." Provide clinical examples of each extreme (too tight, too loose) and describe what balanced collaboration looks like in practice.

Application Across Specialties: Choose your specialty (or intended specialty). Walk through how each of the five domains manifests in your practice. Are all five equally prominent, or do some dominate?

Comparison: How does organizing practice by functional domains (Acute, Chronic, Preventative, Interdisciplinary, Specialty) differ from organizing by tasks or settings? What advantages does the domain approach offer?

Equal Height Columns: The model depicts all five columns as equal height, emphasizing no domain is subordinate. Do you agree all five are equally essential? Could an NP practice autonomously while neglecting one domain?

Evaluation: Some might argue the model is too abstract or theoretical for everyday practice. Others might say it provides essential structure. Which view do you support and why?

Synthesis: Create your own visual representation of how you understand nursopathic medicine. It doesn't have to be architectural, choose whatever metaphor works for you. Explain your choices.

1. INTRODUCTION: A UNIFIED FRAMEWORK

The Nursopathic Medicine Practice Model conceptualizes nurse practitioner practice as a unified system of autonomous clinical authority grounded in advanced nursing judgment. The model is organized around five functional domains that describe how nurse practitioners reason and practice across all specialties, rather than focusing on specific services or tasks.

This chapter presents both the conceptual framework and its visual representation, designed to communicate the structural relationships between domains and their shared foundation. The visual model employs classical Roman architectural metaphors to emphasize the strength, stability, and enduring nature of autonomous nursing practice.

2. THE FIVE DOMAINS

The five domains were identified through analysis of existing advanced practice competency frameworks and role-function literature. National competency standards for nurse practitioners (NONPF, 2017; AACN, 2021) describe what nurse practitioners do in terms of knowledge areas and performance expectations. Bryant-Lukosius and DiCenso (2004) proposed a framework for evaluating advanced practice roles organized around the clinical activities those roles perform. Hamric et al. (2014) identified core competencies that cut across all advanced practice nursing roles, including direct care, ethical decision-making, and collaborative practice. When these competency frameworks are examined not by knowledge domain but by the type of clinical activity involved (episodic response to acute conditions, sustained management of chronic conditions, proactive risk reduction, engagement with other disciplines, and application of population- or condition-specific expertise) five functional domains emerge. These are the domains this model describes. They are not invented categories but a reorganization of documented practice activity into a structure that reflects how autonomous diagnostic-therapeutic practice actually functions across the patient encounter.

The model consists of five domains, each representing a distinct yet interconnected dimension of autonomous practice:

- **Acute Care** encompasses episodic assessment, diagnostic reasoning, and timely intervention in response to emergent, destabilizing, or time-sensitive conditions. Within this domain, nurse practitioners synthesize clinical data, generate working diagnoses, and initiate treatment independently within scope.
- **Chronic Care** reflects sustained responsibility for monitoring treatment response, adjusting interventions, and managing outcomes over time. This domain emphasizes continuity, accountability, and the iterative refinement of clinical decisions as patient conditions evolve.
- **Preventative Care** integrates risk assessment, screening, anticipatory guidance, and health promotion when clinically

appropriate. Rather than representing a discrete service line, this domain reflects the professional obligation of nurse practitioners to reduce risk, prevent deterioration, and optimize functional outcomes across all practice settings.

- **Interdisciplinary Care** represents the nurse practitioner's engagement with other healthcare disciplines to enhance patient outcomes while maintaining autonomous clinical authority. This domain acknowledges that modern healthcare requires collaboration with allopathic and osteopathic physicians, pharmacists, physical therapists, psychologists, dentists, and other professionals, while preserving independent decision-making responsibility within nursing scope.
- **Specialty Care** encompasses population- or condition-focused expertise that informs advanced assessment, diagnosis, and management within defined clinical domains. This domain allows the model to remain inclusive of diverse specialties while maintaining a unified theoretical structure.

3. FOUNDATION: EVIDENCE-BASED PRACTICE

These five domains rest upon a shared foundation of **Evidence-Based Practice**, affirming that autonomous authority is exercised within established scientific and professional standards. Evidence-based practice ensures that clinical decisions are informed by current research, clinical guidelines, and professional consensus while remaining individualized to patient context.

4. VISUAL REPRESENTATION: THE ARCHITECTURAL MODEL

The Nursopathic Medicine Practice Model is represented visually through classical Roman architectural elements, a design choice that conveys stability, timelessness, and structural integrity. This visual metaphor serves both pedagogical and conceptual purposes, making the abstract relationships between domains concrete and memorable.

The Structure

- **The Pediment (Roof):** At the apex of the structure sits a triangular pediment bearing the inscription "NURSOPATHIC MEDICINE" in gold lettering. This placement signifies that the five domains, when integrated and supported by evidence-based practice, constitute nursopathic medicine itself. The pediment represents the unified whole that emerges from the structural elements below. The gold inscription conveys the enduring value and excellence of the framework.

  The Entablature: Immediately below the pediment, a horizontal entablature in white marble bears the inscription "AUTONOMOUS NURSE PRACTITIONER PRACTICE" in gold lettering and provides structural unity across all five columns. This element symbolizes the coherence of the framework, that despite representing distinct functional domains, all five contribute to a single professional model.
- **The Five Columns:** Each domain is represented as a classical Corinthian column of equal height and prominence, crafted in white marble. The choice of equal-height columns is deliberate: no domain is subordinate to another; all are essential to autonomous practice. The white marble represents the purity, strength, and timeless nature of professional nursing practice. The columns are:
    1. **Acute Care** (First column)
    2. **Chronic Care** (Second column)
    3. **Preventative Care** (Third column)
    4. **Interdisciplinary Care** (Fourth column) - Distinguished by a green vine
    5. **Specialty Care** (Fifth column)

  Each column features classical architectural elements:
    - **Corinthian Capitals:** Ornate tops representing the refined nature of advanced practice expertise

- **Fluted Shafts:** Vertical grooves in white marble symbolizing strength through structure and the disciplined application of clinical reasoning
- **Attic Bases:** Multi-tiered bases suggesting the developmental progression from education through professional formation to autonomous practice
- **The Green Vine of Unity:** The Interdisciplinary Care column is distinguished by a graceful green vine spiraling up its shaft, adorned with leaves. This vine carries profound symbolic meaning:

The vine represents unity in collaboration, the organic, living connection between nurse practitioners and other healthcare disciplines. The spiraling pattern illustrates that collaboration winds throughout practice, touching all aspects of care. Critically, the vine's measured spiral conveys balance: too tight a grip constricts care, limiting flexibility and suffocating autonomous judgment; too loose a hold fumbles care, allowing fragmentation and poor coordination.

The vine must be present but not strangling, supportive but not restrictive, visible but not dominating. This visual metaphor captures the essence of Interdisciplinary Care within nursopathic medicine: collaboration that enhances rather than constrains, unifies rather than subordinates, and strengthens rather than weakens autonomous practice. The green color symbolizes growth, vitality, and the organic nature of professional relationships.

The Stylobate (Foundation): All five columns rest upon a substantial stepped platform of white marble bearing the inscription "EVIDENCE-BASED PRACTICE" in gold. This foundation represents the scientific and professional standards that support and legitimize autonomous authority. The stepped design suggests layers of evidence (research, guidelines, clinical consensus, and professional standards) upon which all domains depend. The gold inscription emphasizes that evidence-based practice is the precious, enduring principle underlying all autonomous authority.

5. INTERPRETING THE ARCHITECTURAL METAPHOR

The architectural metaphor is not merely decorative; it conveys essential conceptual relationships:

- **Structural Interdependence:** Just as Roman temples required all columns to support the roof, autonomous practice requires all five domains functioning together. Removing any domain would compromise the integrity of the whole structure.
- **Equal Importance:** The equal height of all columns emphasizes that nurse practitioners must develop competence across all five domains. Expertise in Acute Care without Preventative Care, or Specialty Care without Interdisciplinary Care, represents incomplete professional development.
- **Material Unity:** The white marble construction across all columns represents the unified professional identity of nurse practitioners. Despite different domains, all practice occurs within the same framework, guided by the same nursing values, and accountable to the same professional standards.
- **The Vine's Lesson:** The green vine on the Interdisciplinary Care column teaches a critical lesson about collaboration. Healthy interdisciplinary relationships are like well-tended vines: they grow organically, provide support without constriction, and enhance the structure without overwhelming it. Too much control. Vines wound too tightly, strangles autonomous practice and creates dependency. Too little coordination, vines hanging loosely, allows fragmentation and poor patient outcomes. The balanced vine illustrates the ideal: present, supportive, organic, but not dominating.
- **Gold as Excellence:** The gold inscriptions for "NURSOPATHIC MEDICINE" and "EVIDENCE-BASED PRACTICE" signify that these principles are precious and enduring. Gold does not tarnish or fade; similarly, these foundational commitments remain constant even as practice environments change.
- **Foundational Support:** The prominence of the Evidence-Based Practice foundation emphasizes that autonomy

is never arbitrary or unaccountable. All clinical authority rests upon scientific and professional standards.

- **Permanence and Stability:** Classical architecture evokes timelessness and durability. This visual choice signals that nursopathic medicine is not a temporary adaptation or expedient solution, but a stable, enduring framework for understanding autonomous nursing practice.
- **Professional Dignity:** The classical aesthetic conveys gravitas and professional seriousness, reflecting the weight of responsibility that accompanies autonomous clinical authority. The use of white marble (associated with monuments, temples, and enduring structures) suggests that nurse practitioner practice deserves to be understood as substantial, permanent, and worthy of respect.

6. MODEL STRUCTURE AND FUNCTION

The functional design of the model allows direct application across all nurse practitioner roles. Rather than defining practice by setting or task, the model describes the reasoning processes and responsibilities that characterize autonomous practice in any context.

The visual model serves as an organizing framework for understanding how these functional domains operate:

- **Vertically:** Each column represents depth of practice within a domain, from foundational competence through advanced expertise.
- **Horizontally:** The entablature represents integration across domains, reminding practitioners that clinical situations rarely isolate within a single domain.
- **Foundationally:** Evidence-based practice grounds all domains, ensuring that autonomy remains accountable and scientifically justified.

7. APPLICATION ACROSS SPECIALTIES

In psychiatric practice, Acute Care includes crisis evaluation and stabilization, while Chronic Care reflects ongoing psychopharmacologic and therapeutic management. Preventative Care encompasses relapse prevention and mitigation of treatment-related risks. Interdisciplinary Care involves collaboration with psychiatrists, psychologists, social workers, and primary care providers. Specialty Care is expressed through psychiatric expertise and population-focused knowledge.

In acute care settings, the same domains apply through rapid diagnostic reasoning (Acute Care), inpatient condition management (Chronic Care), complication prevention (Preventative Care), team-based coordination (Interdisciplinary Care), and critical care expertise (Specialty Care).

In primary care, family nurse practitioners engage in urgent problem evaluation (Acute Care), chronic disease management (Chronic Care), health maintenance and screening (Preventative Care), referral and consultation (Interdisciplinary Care), and lifespan-focused practice (Specialty Care).

The visual model reinforces this universal applicability. Regardless of specialty, the five columns remain constant. What varies is the specific expression of each domain within different populations and contexts.

8. PEDAGOGICAL APPLICATIONS OF THE MODEL

The visual model serves multiple educational purposes:

- **Curriculum Organization:** Educational programs can structure learning objectives, clinical experiences, and competency assessments around the five domains, ensuring systematic development of autonomous practice capacity.
- **Professional Identity Formation:** The model provides students with a clear, memorable image of what it means to practice as a nurse practitioner. The architectural metaphor

helps learners understand that they are building something substantial and enduring.

- **Clinical Reasoning Framework:** In clinical settings, the five-column structure offers a mental checklist: Am I considering acute needs? Chronic management? Prevention? Interdisciplinary resources? Specialty-specific factors?
- **Assessment and Evaluation:** Faculty and preceptors can evaluate student progress across all five domains, identifying strengths and areas requiring further development before graduation.
- **Lifelong Learning:** Practicing nurse practitioners can use the model for self-assessment and continuing education planning, ensuring ongoing competence across all domains.

9. REGULATORY AND PROFESSIONAL APPLICATIONS

The model also serves regulatory and professional functions:

- **Scope Definition:** By describing functional domains rather than task lists, the model provides a flexible yet rigorous framework for defining scope of practice that adapts to evolving healthcare needs.
- **Competency Standards:** Certification bodies and regulatory agencies can use the five domains as organizing principles for competency assessment, ensuring thorough evaluation of autonomous practice readiness.
- **Public Communication:** The visual model offers a clear, accessible way to explain nurse practitioner practice to patients, policymakers, and other stakeholders. The architectural metaphor communicates strength, stability, and accountability.
- **Interdisciplinary Dialogue:** By explicitly including Interdisciplinary Care as a domain, the model signals to other professions that collaboration is integral to nursopathic medicine rather than incidental or conditional.

10. DURABILITY AND COHERENCE

The model's strength lies in its durability across specialties and settings. By organizing practice around functional domains rather than tasks or environments, it provides a stable framework that accommodates the diversity of nurse practitioner roles while maintaining professional coherence.

As practice environments continue to evolve, new specialties emerge, and healthcare delivery models change, the five-domain structure remains applicable. The columns may bear different weights in different contexts, but all five remain essential to autonomous practice.

11. EMPLOYMENT SETTINGS AND DOMAIN UTILIZATION

A common question arises: What about nurse practitioners whose employment settings emphasize some domains more than others? An NP working in an urgent care clinic may see primarily episodic acute presentations with limited opportunity for longitudinal chronic disease management. An NP working in a specialty consultation role may focus heavily on Specialty Care and Interdisciplinary Care with less emphasis on Preventative Care. Does the model still apply?

The answer is yes, and the distinction is critical: the five domains describe what nurse practitioners are educated and certified to do, not necessarily what every employment setting requires them to do daily. Scope of practice is determined by education, certification, and licensure. Not by employment setting. An NP working in urgent care retains the full scope of practice for which they are certified, even if that particular role does not require daily use of all five domains.

Consider three examples:

11.1 Urgent Care NP:

This role emphasizes Acute Care (episodic problem evaluation). However, the NP still engages Preventative Care (identifying risk factors and providing anticipatory guidance even in brief encounters), Interdisciplinary Care (consulting when presentations exceed scope or warrant specialty input), and Specialty Care (applying population-specific knowledge to presenting problems). Chronic Care may be limited to recognizing uncontrolled conditions and facilitating appropriate follow-up. The domains are all present, even if Acute Care dominates the daily workflow.

11.2 Specialty Consultation NP:

A cardiology NP may focus primarily on Specialty Care (cardiovascular expertise) and Interdisciplinary Care (coordinating with referring providers). However, when evaluating a patient with new chest pain, the NP engages Acute Care. When managing a patient with heart failure over time, the NP engages Chronic Care. When counseling on cardiac risk reduction, the NP engages Preventative Care. Employment in a specialty setting does not eliminate the other domains, it shifts their relative emphasis.

11.3 Primary Care NP:

A family nurse practitioner in a primary care setting engages all five domains regularly and visibly. Acute Care during sick visits, Chronic Care in disease management, Preventative Care through health maintenance and screening, Interdisciplinary Care through referrals and consultations, and Specialty Care through lifespan-focused expertise. This setting may showcase the full model most clearly, but it does not mean other settings use a "reduced" version of the model.

The equal-height columns in the visual model reflect this principle: all five domains are equally essential to autonomous practice, regardless of employment setting. A column does not shrink because it is used less frequently. An NP whose role emphasizes one or two domains remains accountable for competency across all five, because autonomous practice authority is comprehensive, it is not subdivided by employment role.

This distinction has practical implications. When an urgent care NP encounters a patient with poorly controlled diabetes, the NP's responsibility is not to say "I only do acute care." The responsibility is to assess the acute presentation, recognize the chronic disease management gap, provide appropriate interim guidance (Preventative Care), and facilitate appropriate follow-up (Interdisciplinary Care). The employment setting shapes workflow emphasis, but it does not define scope.

Similarly, an NP cannot claim exemption from accountability in one domain because their employment emphasizes others. A cardiology NP who fails to recognize and address an acute presentation because "I'm a specialty consultant" has not practiced within the standards of autonomous practice. The five domains describe the full scope for which the NP is educated, certified, and accountable. Not a menu from which employment settings select portions.

12. VISUAL MODEL SUMMARY

The Nursopathic Medicine Practice Model, represented through classical Roman architecture, consists of:

- **Five equal columns** representing Acute Care, Chronic Care, Preventative Care, Interdisciplinary Care, and Specialty Care
- **A triangular pediment** inscribed with "Nursopathic Medicine," symbolizing the unified framework
- **An entablature** providing horizontal integration across domains
- **A stylobate foundation** inscribed with "Evidence-Based Practice," supporting all domains

This visual representation is not merely illustrative but constitutive, it defines the structural relationships that make nursopathic medicine coherent as a theoretical framework.

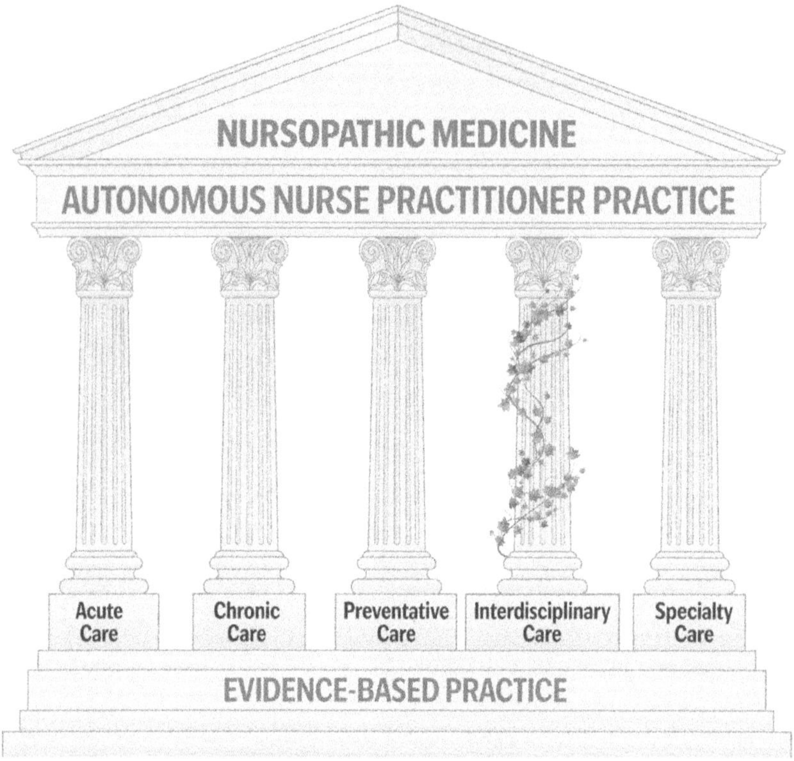

Figure 7.1. The Nursopathic Medicine Practice Model employs classical Roman architectural elements to represent the five functional domains of autonomous nurse practitioner practice. Each domain is depicted as a Corinthian column of equal height crafted in white marble, emphasizing that all domains are equally essential and unified within nursing's professional identity. The columns rest upon a foundation of Evidence-Based Practice and support the unified structure of Nursopathic Medicine, both inscribed in gold to convey enduring excellence. The Interdisciplinary Care column features a green vine symbolizing unity in collaboration, balanced to neither constrict care through excessive control nor fumble it through insufficient coordination. The architectural metaphor conveys stability, permanence, structural integrity, and the organic nature of professional collaboration.

CHAPTER SUMMARY

The Nursopathic Medicine Practice Model organizes autonomous nurse practitioner practice into five functional domains (Acute Care, Chronic Care, Preventative Care, Interdisciplinary Care, and Specialty Care) supported by a foundation of evidence-based practice. The visual representation employs classical Roman architectural elements to convey structural relationships, stability, and professional dignity. This structure provides a unified framework applicable across all specialties and settings, emphasizing reasoning and accountability rather than tasks or locations. The model serves pedagogical, regulatory, and professional communication functions while maintaining conceptual coherence across the diversity of nurse practitioner roles.

CHAPTER 7
PRACTICE QUESTIONS

MULTIPLE CHOICE QUESTIONS

1. **The Nursopathic Medicine Practice Model consists of:**
   A. Three domains
   B. Five domains
   C. Seven competencies
   D. Ten standards

2. **The five domains are:**
   A. Assessment, Diagnosis, Planning, Implementation, Evaluation
   B. Acute Care, Chronic Care, Preventative Care, Interdisciplinary Care, Specialty Care
   C. Primary, Secondary, Tertiary, Quaternary, Quinary
   D. Novice, Advanced Beginner, Competent, Proficient, Expert

3. **All five domains rest upon a foundation of:**
   A. Physician collaboration
   B. Hospital policies
   C. Evidence-Based Practice
   D. Institutional accreditation

4. **The architectural model uses which classical style?**
   A. Greek
   B. Roman
   C. Gothic
   D. Modern

5. **What does the white marble in the visual model represent?**
   A. Purity, strength, and timeless nature of professional nursing
   B. Cost of education
   C. Hospital environment
   D. Medical authority

6. **The green vine on the Interdisciplinary Care column symbolizes:**
   A. Environmental health
   B. Unity in collaboration, balanced to neither constrict nor fumble care
   C. Natural healing
   D. Organic food recommendations

7. **The equal height of all five columns emphasizes:**
   A. All patients are equal
   B. No domain is subordinate, all are equally essential
   C. All NPs earn the same salary
   D. All specialties are identical

8. **When the vine is "too tight" it:**
   A. Provides needed support
   B. Constricts care and limits autonomous judgment
   C. Improves patient outcomes
   D. Strengthens the structure

9. **The model is organized around functional domains rather than:**
   A. Evidence
   B. Specific tasks or settings
   C. Patient populations
   D. Educational requirements

10. A psychiatric NP applies the five domains through:

A. Different domains than other specialties

B. Crisis evaluation (Acute), ongoing management (Chronic), relapse prevention (Preventative), consultation with other disciplines (Interdisciplinary), and psychiatric population expertise (Specialty)

C. Only Specialty Care

D. Only Acute Care

11. An NP working in urgent care sees primarily episodic acute presentations. This means:

A. The other four domains do not apply to their practice

B. They are only accountable for Acute Care competency

C. Employment setting determines which domains are used most frequently, but all five remain part of their scope and accountability

D. Their certification scope is reduced to match their employment role

CASE-BASED APPLICATION QUESTIONS

Case Scenario 1:

You're presenting the nursopathic medicine model to a group of NP students who find the architectural metaphor confusing. They ask, "Why columns and vines? Why not just a list of what we do?"

Questions:

- Explain why the architectural metaphor is used rather than a simple list.
- What does the structural interdependence (all columns supporting the roof) teach that a list cannot?
- How does the visual model aid in professional identity formation?

Case Scenario 2:

An NP working in an urgent care clinic says, "I only see episodic acute presentations. I don't manage chronic diseases longitudinally and I rarely do preventive care beyond routine screenings. Does the five-domain model really apply to my practice, or is it just for primary care?"

Questions:

- Using the equal-height columns concept, how would you respond to this NP?
- Provide concrete examples of how an urgent care NP engages all five domains even when Acute Care dominates the workflow.
- Explain the difference between employment setting and scope of practice. Why does this distinction matter for accountability?

TRUE/FALSE SELF-ASSESSMENT

6. ______ The model consists of three domains.
7. ______ All five domains rest on Evidence-Based Practice foundation.
8. ______ The green vine symbolizes unity in collaboration.
9. ______ When the vine is too tight, it provides appropriate structure.
10. ______ The model is organized by specific tasks rather than functional domains.

See Appendix B for complete answers and rationales.

PART III

THE FIVE DOMAINS OF PRACTICE

CHAPTER 8

ACUTE CARE

LEARNING OBJECTIVES

Upon completing this chapter, students will be able to:

Define the Acute Care domain and explain its scope across specialties and settings.

Describe clinical reasoning under time constraints, including pattern recognition and probabilistic reasoning.

Analyze how NPs determine thresholds for action (intervention vs. observation, escalation vs. stabilization).

Explain accountability for outcomes in acute clinical decision-making.

Apply acute care principles to diverse specialty contexts (family, psychiatric, acute care, pediatric, etc.).

Evaluate when acute decision-making requires consultation versus independent management.

Integrate Acute Care with other domains (chronic exacerbations, preventative aspects, interdisciplinary needs).

CRITICAL THINKING QUESTIONS

Application: Compare acute clinical decision-making in three different settings: emergency department (AGACNP), psychiatric crisis (PMHNP), and urgent care (FNP). What's similar? What differs?

Risk Assessment: You're managing a patient with chest pain. Walk through your threshold determination process: What factors push you toward immediate intervention? Toward observation? Toward consultation or referral?

Analysis: The chapter states that in acute care, "decisions are often made with incomplete data." How does nursopathic medicine prepare NPs to manage this uncertainty responsibly? What distinguishes responsible uncertainty management from recklessness?

Comparison: How does the Acute Care domain in nursopathic medicine differ from emergency medicine practiced by physicians? What makes it nursing-centered?

Integration: Provide an example where acute decision-making intersects with at least two other domains. How do you manage these overlapping needs?

Evaluation: The chapter emphasizes that Acute Care is defined by "assumption of responsibility under conditions of uncertainty" rather than by setting. Do you find this definition useful? Why or why not?

Reflection: Describe a time you (or an NP you observed) made an acute clinical decision. Analyze that decision using the framework from this chapter: What reasoning was used? How was accountability demonstrated?

1. PURPOSE AND SCOPE

Acute Care represents a foundational domain of autonomous nurse practitioner practice. This domain encompasses the capacity to rapidly assess, synthesize clinical information, establish working diagnoses, and initiate timely interventions in response to emergent, unstable, or time-sensitive conditions. The defining feature of this domain is not the setting in which care occurs, but the assumption of responsibility for clinical outcomes under conditions of uncertainty.

Within nursopathic medicine, acute decision-making is understood as an expression of advanced nursing judgment rather than a discrete set of tasks. It reflects the nurse practitioner's ability to integrate evidence, clinical experience, and patient context to act decisively while remaining accountable for consequences. The clinical reasoning methods that underpin this domain—particularly acute reasoning—are grounded in the five methods of clinical reasoning established in Chapter 4, which provides the intellectual foundation for all five domains of practice.

2. CLINICAL REASONING UNDER TIME CONSTRAINTS

Acute clinical environments compress time, increase risk, and limit information. In this context, nurse practitioners rely on pattern recognition, prioritization, and probabilistic reasoning to guide action (Croskerry, 2002). Decisions are often made with incomplete data and must balance immediacy against safety.

This reasoning process is iterative rather than linear. Initial assessments generate provisional diagnoses that are refined as new information emerges. The nurse practitioner's authority lies not in certainty, but in the capacity to manage uncertainty responsibly.

3. RISK ASSESSMENT AND THRESHOLDS FOR ACTION

A central feature of acute decision-making is the determination of thresholds for intervention. Nurse practitioners must continuously evaluate the risk of action versus inaction, escalation versus stabilization, and independent management versus collaboration.

These thresholds are shaped by clinical presentation, patient vulnerability, available resources, and professional accountability. Within nursopathic medicine, the authority to act includes the responsibility to recognize limits and to initiate appropriate escalation when warranted.

4. ACCOUNTABILITY AND OUTCOME RESPONSIBILITY

Autonomous acute decision-making carries explicit accountability for patient outcomes. Nurse practitioners practicing within this domain are responsible for the rationale underlying decisions, the appropriateness of interventions, and the timeliness of reassessment.

Documentation in acute contexts serves not only legal or institutional purposes, but also reflects professional reasoning. Clear articulation of assessment, decision pathways, and response to change reinforces transparency and accountability.

5. INTEGRATION WITH OTHER DOMAINS

Acute Care does not exist in isolation. It intersects with Chronic Care when acute exacerbations occur in patients with ongoing conditions, with Preventative Care through secondary prevention of complications, with Interdisciplinary Care when consultation or referral is indicated, and with Specialty Care when population-specific expertise guides acute management.

6. DURABILITY ACROSS SETTINGS AND SPECIALTIES

Acute clinical decision-making is not confined to emergency departments or inpatient units. It occurs wherever patient stability can change rapidly, including outpatient clinics, psychiatric settings, and specialty practices. The durability of this domain across contexts reinforces its role as a structural pillar of autonomous practice.

7. ILLUSTRATIVE EXAMPLES ACROSS SPECIALTIES

- **Family NP:** Rapid assessment and stabilization of undifferentiated acute presentations in ambulatory care, such as acute respiratory distress, chest pain, or abdominal pain requiring immediate diagnostic reasoning.
- **Adult-Gerontology Acute Care NP:** Diagnostic and therapeutic decisions for unstable hospitalized patients, including management of sepsis, respiratory failure, or acute decompensation of chronic conditions.
- **Psychiatric-Mental Health NP:** Crisis evaluation, risk stratification for suicide or violence, and initiation of stabilization strategies in acute psychiatric presentations.

- **Pediatric NP:** Acute illness assessment and intervention incorporating developmental considerations, such as fever evaluation, dehydration management, or respiratory distress in children.
- **Neonatal NP:** Immediate clinical decision-making for physiologic instability in neonatal populations, including resuscitation and management of prematurity complications.
- **Women's Health NP:** Acute gynecologic or obstetric evaluation requiring timely intervention, such as ectopic pregnancy, severe preeclampsia, or acute pelvic infections.

8. CASE STUDIES

8.1 Case A: Acute Care in Primary Care Setting

- **Case Presentation:**

  Maria Gonzalez, FNP, is working in a busy community health center when a 58-year-old male patient, Mr. James Patterson, arrives as a walk-in with chest discomfort that began 30 minutes ago. The medical assistant brings him directly to an exam room and alerts Maria.
- **Initial Assessment (2 minutes):**

  Chief complaint: "Pressure in my chest, feels heavy"

  Vital signs: BP 168/94, HR 102, RR 20, O2 sat 94% on room air, temp 98.4°F

  Appears diaphoretic, clutching chest, anxious

  Medical history: Hypertension (not well-controlled), type 2 diabetes, hyperlipidemia, 40 pack-year smoking history
- **Acute Clinical Reasoning Under Time Constraints:**

  Maria immediately recognizes this as a potentially life-threatening presentation requiring rapid decision-making. Her pattern recognition triggers acute coronary syndrome (ACS) protocols while she simultaneously considers differential diagnoses.

  Within 5 minutes, Maria:

Calls EMS – Recognizes need for emergent transport rather than delaying for complete workup

Initiates interventions:

- Aspirin 324 mg chewed
- Sublingual nitroglycerin 0.4 mg (after confirming no phosphodiesterase inhibitor use)
- Oxygen via nasal cannula to maintain O2 sat >94%
- IV access established

Obtains 12-lead EKG – Shows ST elevations in leads II, III, aVF (inferior STEMI)

Calls receiving hospital – Activates cardiac catheterization lab, provides report

Documents critical decision points and interventions with time stamps

Communicates with patient and family about transfer and prognosis

- **Integration with Other Domains:**

  Chronic Care: Maria recognizes this acute event in context of poorly controlled chronic conditions

  Preventative Care: Missed opportunity for more aggressive risk reduction now becomes secondary prevention focus

  Interdisciplinary Care: Seamless handoff to EMS, emergency department, and cardiology

  Specialty Care: Recognizes limits, needs cardiology intervention, not within NP scope to manage STEMI definitively

- **Accountability and Outcome:**

  Maria's rapid recognition, appropriate interventions, and timely transfer potentially saved Mr. Patterson's life. She demonstrated autonomous decision-making under extreme time pressure while maintaining clear accountability. Her documentation reflected her clinical reasoning: why aspirin and nitroglycerine immediately, why EMS rather than private transport, why cath lab activation was urgent.

- **Discussion Questions:**
    1. What specific aspects of Maria's reasoning demonstrated autonomous practice?
    2. How did time constraints affect her decision-making process?
    3. At what point did she determine this required emergent transfer rather than clinic management?
    4. How did she balance autonomy with appropriate escalation?
    5. What would have happened if she had delayed to "get more information" or "call the collaborating physician"?

8.2 Case B: Acute Care in Psychiatric Setting

- **Case Presentation:**

  David Chen, PMHNP, is covering the adult inpatient psychiatric unit when he's called to assess a 32-year-old female patient, Ms. Sarah Miller, admitted three days ago for major depressive disorder with suicidal ideation. Nursing staff report she's become increasingly agitated, pacing, and stating "I need to leave now, they're coming for me."

- **Initial Assessment (Immediate):**

  Mental status: Agitated, paranoid, disorganized thought process

  Speech: Pressured, tangential

  Perceptual disturbances: "I hear them telling me what to do"

  Vital signs: BP 148/92, HR 118, RR 22

  No history of psychotic disorder in chart

  Recent medication changes: Bupropion started 48 hours ago

- **Acute Clinical Reasoning in Psychiatric Emergency:**

  David recognizes this as an acute change requiring immediate assessment for safety and potential medical causes. His differential includes:

- Bupropion-induced psychosis (drug-related)
- Underlying bipolar disorder with psychotic features (now unmasked)
- Medical condition causing delirium (infection, metabolic, neurologic)
- Rapid cycling or mixed episode
- Substance intoxication (though toxicology was negative on admission)

Within 15 minutes, David:

Ensures safety – Staff maintaining constant observation, environment secured

Holds bupropion – Recognizes potential medication-induced psychosis

Orders stat labs – CBC, CMP, urinalysis to rule out infection/ metabolic causes

Initiates pharmacologic intervention:

- Olanzapine 10 mg IM for acute agitation and emerging psychosis
- Lorazepam 2 mg IM for agitation and anxiety

Arranges medical consultation – Requests internal medicine evaluation given acute change

Reassesses every 30 minutes for response and side effects

Documents thoroughly including differential diagnosis, reasoning, interventions, and monitoring plan

Communicates with patient (as she stabilizes), family, and treatment team

- **Integration with Other Domains:**

  Chronic Care: Recognizes this changes long-term diagnosis and treatment approach

  Preventative Care: Secondary prevention, preventing harm during acute crisis

  Interdisciplinary Care: Collaborates with medicine to rule out organic causes

Specialty Care: Uses psychiatric expertise to differentiate psychiatric emergency from medical emergency

- **Outcome and Accountability:**

  Sarah stabilized within 2 hours. Medical workup revealed UTI contributing to acute mental status change. David's comprehensive differential and willingness to hold psychotropic medication that might be causative, combined with appropriate medical consultation, prevented misdiagnosis. His autonomous decision to medicate for safety while simultaneously investigating organic causes reflected sophisticated clinical reasoning.

- **Discussion Questions:**

  1. How did David balance urgent safety needs with diagnostic uncertainty?
  2. What role did his psychiatric specialty expertise play in recognizing this as atypical?
  3. How did holding the bupropion demonstrate autonomous clinical judgment?
  4. What might have happened with delayed or inadequate response?
  5. How did David integrate medical and psychiatric reasoning?

Clinical Reflection: Racing Mind, Racing Clock

Throughout my years in autonomous psychiatric practice, I have encountered acute clinical situations that demanded rapid assessment, careful risk stratification, and decisive medication management—often without the luxury of complete information. One case stands out as a clear illustration of what acute clinical reasoning looks like from the inside.

The patient was referred to me by a close LMHC colleague with whom I have a long-standing professional relationship built on mutual trust and shared clinical values. We refer patients to each other regularly—she handles the psychotherapeutic work; I manage the pharmacologic side. When she sends me someone, I take it seriously. This patient arrived with five nights of virtually no sleep, severe mood swings, escalating irritability, and a family environment that had deteriorated into open conflict. The clinical picture was consistent with acute bipolar mania requiring immediate intervention.

What complicated the picture was her history of alcoholism. She had been sober for two months—a meaningful but relatively brief window—which introduced real uncertainty about her hepatic status. Valproic acid (Depakote), my preferred mood stabilizer in acute bipolar mania, carries the risk of elevating liver enzymes, and in a patient with alcohol history that risk is not theoretical. I could not simply proceed as I would with an otherwise healthy patient.

My reasoning unfolded in real time. I made two decisions simultaneously. First, I started Depakote at a conservative dose, lower than I would typically use, to account for the hepatic uncertainty. This was a deliberate calibration—not avoiding the medication, but respecting the incomplete picture. Second, I added Olanzapine at a higher starting dose. Olanzapine served a dual purpose: it would bring the acute manic symptoms down faster than a mood stabilizer alone could achieve, providing the rapid stabilization she needed while the Depakote built toward therapeutic effect.

Together, the two medications addressed both the urgency of her presentation and the clinical caution her history required.

I also ordered baseline labs at the first visit. Not because I could wait for results before treating—the presentation was too acute for that—but because establishing a baseline immediately would allow me to interpret any subsequent changes in context. This is anticipatory reasoning embedded within acute management: acting now while creating the data infrastructure to evaluate what comes next.

That night, I did not sleep well. I lay awake running through the decision. Had I calibrated the Depakote dose correctly? Was the Olanzapine dose sufficient to bring her down before she escalated further or harmed a relationship she couldn't repair? The next morning I texted my LMHC colleague—not to discuss the medication, which is outside her role as a therapist, but simply to tell her that I hadn't slept because I was worried about her patient. That text was not a clinical consultation. It was one clinician telling another: I received the trust you placed in me, and I am carrying it. That kind of accountability—felt personally, not just professionally—is part of what autonomous practice means.

The patient was compliant. Within a couple of days she had returned to baseline. Her labs, when they came back, showed normal liver enzymes—the hepatic risk I had been managing carefully had not materialized. She has since expressed profound gratitude for how quickly her symptoms were addressed.

> *What this case illustrates is precisely what the Acute Care domain describes: clinical decision-making made under conditions of genuine uncertainty, without the luxury of waiting for complete information, with full accountability for the outcome. I did not know her liver enzymes were normal when I started Depakote. I acted on the best available clinical reasoning—conservative dosing, a bridging agent, immediate baseline labs—and monitored closely. That is what autonomous acute practice requires. Not certainty. Judgment in the absence of certainty, accompanied by the responsibility to watch carefully for what you could not yet know.*

CHAPTER SUMMARY

Acute Care within nursopathic medicine reflects the nurse practitioner's capacity to act decisively, responsibly, and autonomously under conditions of uncertainty. By framing acute care as a function of reasoning and accountability rather than location or task, this domain reinforces the legitimacy and durability of autonomous nursing practice across specialties. Clinical authority in this domain is exercised through rapid assessment, risk evaluation, and outcome responsibility.

CHAPTER 8
PRACTICE QUESTIONS

MULTIPLE CHOICE QUESTIONS

1. **The Acute Care domain is defined by:**
   A. The setting (emergency department, ICU)
   B. Assumption of responsibility under conditions of uncertainty
   C. Physician supervision
   D. Simple, straightforward cases

2. **Acute Care encompasses:**
   A. Only emergency situations
   B. Episodic assessment, diagnostic reasoning, and timely intervention for time-sensitive conditions
   C. Routine wellness visits
   D. Scheduled surgeries only

3. **Decisions in acute care are often made with:**
   A. Complete information
   B. Incomplete data requiring management of uncertainty
   C. Physician direction
   D. Unlimited time

4. **Pattern recognition in acute care allows NPs to:**
   A. Avoid diagnostic reasoning
   B. Rapidly synthesize clinical information despite time constraints
   C. Delay decision-making
   D. Transfer all care to physicians

5. **Thresholds for action in acute care involve determining:**
   A. Billing codes
   B. Risk of action vs. inaction, escalation vs. stabilization
   C. Patient preferences only
   D. Insurance coverage

6. **Accountability in acute care requires:**
   A. Physician countersignature
   B. Clear articulation of assessment, decision pathways, and response to change
   C. Transferring responsibility to consultants
   D. Avoiding documentation

7. **Acute Care integrates with Chronic Care when:**
   A. Never, they're completely separate
   B. Acute exacerbations occur in patients with ongoing conditions
   C. Only in primary care
   D. Regulations require it

8. **Acute clinical decision-making occurs:**
   A. Only in emergency departments
   B. Wherever patient stability can change rapidly
   C. Only in hospitals
   D. Only during business hours

9. **A PMHNP evaluating a patient with new-onset psychosis is performing:**
   A. Chronic Care only
   B. Acute Care, crisis evaluation and stabilization
   C. Preventative Care
   D. Specialty Care only

10. **The authority to act in acute situations includes responsibility to:**
   A. Always manage independently
   B. Recognize limits and initiate appropriate escalation when warranted
   C. Never consult others
   D. Avoid difficult cases

CASE-BASED APPLICATION QUESTIONS

Case Scenario 1:

Maria, an FNP in a community health center, sees a 58-year-old male with chest pressure that began 30 minutes ago. BP 168/94, HR 102, diaphoretic, anxious. He has hypertension, diabetes, hyperlipidemia, and 40 pack-year smoking history. She immediately recognizes this as potentially life-threatening.

Questions:

- What specific aspects of Maria's immediate response demonstrate autonomous Acute Care practice?
- How does she balance immediate intervention with appropriate escalation?
- What would have been the consequences of delaying to "get more information" or "call the collaborating physician"?

Case Scenario 2:

David, a PMHNP on an inpatient unit, is called to assess Sarah, a 32-year-old admitted three days ago for depression, now acutely agitated, paranoid, with auditory hallucinations. This is a new symptom cluster. Bupropion was started 48 hours ago.

Questions:

- Describe David's differential diagnosis and why it demonstrates comprehensive acute reasoning.
- How does he balance safety needs with diagnostic uncertainty?
- Why was holding the bupropion an example of autonomous clinical judgment?

TRUE/FALSE SELF-ASSESSMENT

1. ______ Acute Care is defined by the setting (ED, ICU) rather than function.
2. ______ Decisions in acute care always require complete information.
3. ______ Pattern recognition is a legitimate form of clinical reasoning in acute contexts.
4. ______ Authority to act includes responsibility to recognize limits and escalate appropriately.
5. ______ Acute Care is incompatible with collaboration.

See Appendix B for complete answers and rationales.

CHAPTER 9

CHRONIC CARE

LEARNING OBJECTIVES

Upon completing this chapter, students will be able to:

Define the Chronic Care domain and explain its emphasis on continuity and longitudinal accountability.

Describe clinical reasoning over time, including pattern recognition across repeated encounters.

Explain the processes of monitoring, adjustment, and outcome evaluation in chronic condition management.

Analyze how NPs maintain continuity across transitions in care settings and intensity.

Apply longitudinal reasoning to diverse chronic conditions and specialty contexts.

Evaluate the relationship between sustained responsibility and therapeutic relationships.

Integrate Chronic Care with acute exacerbations, preventative strategies, and interdisciplinary coordination.

CRITICAL THINKING QUESTIONS

Longitudinal Reasoning: Compare managing acute hypertension (single episode) versus managing chronic hypertension over 10 years. What additional reasoning skills does longitudinal care require?

Application: Choose a chronic condition relevant to your specialty (diabetes, heart failure, depression, COPD, etc.). Map out how the Chronic Care domain functions across 1-2 years of management, including routine visits, adjustments, complications, and successes.

Continuity Challenge: A patient you've managed for years is hospitalized, sees multiple specialists, then returns to your care. How does the Chronic Care domain guide your approach to reintegrating their care?

Analysis: The chapter states that longitudinal accountability requires "deliberate reflection on whether clinical goals are being met." How is this different from episodic accountability? What does it demand of the NP?

Therapeutic Relationship: Explain how the therapeutic relationship in Chronic Care serves as both "a source of clinical insight and a foundation for shared decision-making." Provide specific examples.

Evaluation: Some healthcare systems emphasize brief, episodic encounters over sustained relationships. How does this structural reality challenge the Chronic Care domain? How can NPs maintain longitudinal responsibility despite system constraints?

Synthesis: Design a documentation system or clinical workflow that would specifically support the longitudinal reasoning and continuity emphasized in this chapter. What would it track? How would it prompt reflection?

1. PURPOSE AND SCOPE

Chronic Care represents a core domain of autonomous nurse practitioner practice defined by sustained responsibility for patient care over time. This domain encompasses the ongoing assessment, monitoring, adjustment, and evaluation of treatment plans across the trajectory of illness or wellness. Unlike episodic encounters, Chronic Care is characterized by continuity, accountability, and outcome-focused clinical judgment.

Within nursopathic medicine, Chronic Care reflects advanced nursing authority exercised through iterative decision-making. It requires the nurse practitioner to integrate evolving clinical data, patient response, and contextual factors to refine care plans while maintaining responsibility for long-term outcomes. This iterative process is rooted in the longitudinal reasoning method described in Chapter 4, which establishes how reasoning unfolds across time rather than within a single encounter—making Chapter 4's framework the conceptual foundation upon which this domain builds.

2. CLINICAL REASONING OVER TIME

Longitudinal clinical reasoning unfolds across repeated encounters rather than discrete moments. Nurse practitioners must recognize patterns, trends, and deviations that emerge only through sustained observation. Decisions are informed not only by current presentation, but by the cumulative understanding of patient history, treatment response, and risk trajectory (Benner, 1984).

This form of reasoning emphasizes adaptability. As conditions evolve, initial diagnoses and management strategies may require revision. The nurse practitioner's authority lies in the ability to reassess, recalibrate, and redirect care in response to change.

Table 9.1. Single-Encounter vs. Longitudinal Clinical Reasoning.

Single-Encounter Reasoning	Longitudinal Reasoning
Focus: Today's presentation	**Focus:** Trajectory over time
Data Source: Current visit only	**Data Source:** Accumulated across encounters
Goal: Solve today's problem	**Goal:** Optimize long-term outcomes
Pattern: Episodic, discrete	**Pattern:** Continuous monitoring
Relationship: Transactional	**Relationship:** Therapeutic, sustained
Accountability: This decision	**Accountability:** Cumulative impact over time
Example: "BP high today → Start medication"	**Example:** "BP pattern over 6 months reveals adherence issues → Address barriers, adjust strategy"

3. MONITORING, ADJUSTMENT, AND OUTCOME EVALUATION

A defining feature of Chronic Care is continuous monitoring of therapeutic effectiveness and safety. Nurse practitioners must determine when treatment is effective, when modification is required, and when alternative strategies should be considered.

Outcome evaluation extends beyond symptom control to include functional status, quality of life, and risk mitigation (Bodenheimer & Sinsky, 2014). Longitudinal accountability requires deliberate reflection on whether clinical goals are being met and whether care remains aligned with patient needs and evidence-based standards.

4. CONTINUITY, TRANSITIONS, AND CARE INTEGRATION

Longitudinal responsibility often spans multiple settings, providers, and phases of care. Nurse practitioners play a critical role in maintaining continuity across transitions, including changes in care intensity, location, or team composition.

Within the nursopathic framework, continuity is an active process rather than a passive outcome. It involves intentional communication, coordination, and clinical oversight to preserve coherence in care delivery despite system fragmentation.

5. PROFESSIONAL ACCOUNTABILITY AND THERAPEUTIC RELATIONSHIP

Sustained clinical responsibility deepens professional accountability. Over time, the nurse practitioner assumes responsibility not only for decisions made, but for the cumulative impact of those decisions. This accountability is inseparable from the therapeutic relationship, which serves as both a source of clinical insight and a foundation for shared decision-making.

Longitudinal practice highlights the ethical dimensions of autonomy, including fidelity, transparency, and responsiveness to patient values as conditions change.

6. INTEGRATION WITH OTHER DOMAINS

Chronic Care intersects with Acute Care during exacerbations or complications, with Preventative Care through ongoing risk reduction, with Interdisciplinary Care when coordinating with specialists or other providers, and with Specialty Care when managing population-specific chronic conditions.

7. DURABILITY ACROSS SETTINGS AND SPECIALTIES

Chronic Care occurs across all nurse practitioner specialties, regardless of setting or population. Whether managing chronic disease, psychiatric conditions, recovery trajectories, or specialty-specific care, nurse practitioners exercise autonomous authority through sustained engagement and outcome-oriented reasoning. The durability of this domain reinforces its central role in defining advanced nursing practice.

8. ILLUSTRATIVE EXAMPLES ACROSS SPECIALTIES

- **Family NP:** Ongoing management of chronic medical conditions across the lifespan, such as diabetes, hypertension, asthma, or heart failure with regular monitoring and treatment adjustment.
- **Adult-Gerontology Primary Care NP:** Long-term care planning and monitoring for aging populations, including management of multiple comorbidities and functional decline prevention.
- **Psychiatric-Mental Health NP:** Sustained psychopharmacologic management and symptom trajectory monitoring for conditions such as major depression, bipolar disorder, or schizophrenia.
- **Pediatric NP:** Longitudinal management of chronic childhood conditions such as asthma, ADHD, or developmental disorders with family-centered care coordination.
- **Women's Health NP:** Reproductive and hormonal health management over time, including menopause management, chronic pelvic pain, or endometriosis.

- **Oncology NP:** Long-term treatment monitoring, survivorship care, and management of late effects following cancer therapy.
- **Cardiology NP:** Chronic cardiovascular disease management with outcome tracking, including heart failure monitoring and post-cardiac event secondary prevention.

9. CASE STUDIES

Case 1: Chronic Care Over Five Years

- **Case Presentation:**

  Jennifer Martinez, AGPCNP, has been managing Mrs. Eleanor Davis, now 72 years old, for five years. This case illustrates longitudinal reasoning and sustained accountability.

  Year 1 (Age 67): Initial presentation: New patient, recently relocated to be near daughter. Brings records showing:

  - Hypertension (on lisinopril 10 mg)
  - Prediabetes (HbA1c 5.9%)
  - Hyperlipidemia (on atorvastatin 20 mg)
  - Mild cognitive complaints ("forgetting names")

  Jennifer's longitudinal approach establishes baseline, develops therapeutic relationship, and creates long-term management plan emphasizing prevention of progression.

  Year 2 (Age 68): HbA1c rises to 6.7%. Rather than immediately starting medication, Jennifer:

  - Explores life changes (daughter's divorce creating stress, less time for meal prep)
  - Refers to diabetes education and nutrition counseling
  - Implements shared decision-making about lifestyle vs. medication
  - Monitors quarterly rather than usual 6-month intervals
  - Adjusts based on patient's preference to "try lifestyle changes first"

Year 3 (Age 69): Despite lifestyle efforts, HbA1c now 7.2%. Jennifer:

- Revisits goals of care conversation
- Initiates metformin with careful monitoring (patient reluctant about medications)
- Continues emphasis on nutrition and activity
- Monitors for metformin tolerance and effectiveness
- Adjusts statinfor primary prevention given new diabetes diagnosis
- Notes subtle progression in cognitive complaints, orders MoCA (score: 24/30)

Year 4 (Age 70): Mrs. Davis experiences minor stroke (TIA). Jennifer:

- Intensifies secondary prevention (adds aspirin, optimizes statin)
- Re-evaluates all chronic disease targets in light of stroke risk
- Coordinates with neurology for stroke workup
- Adds SGLT2 inhibitor for cardiovascular benefit in diabetes
- Addresses post-TIA anxiety affecting medication adherence
- Arranges neuropsychology evaluation for cognitive changes

Year 5 (Age 72): Current status:

- Diabetes: HbA1c 6.8% (acceptable for age/comorbidity)
- Blood pressure: 132/78 (acceptable for patient)
- Cognition: MCI diagnosis, on cholinesterase inhibitor, stable
- Functional status: Independent, driving restricted after TIA
- Quality of life: Good despite chronic conditions

- **Longitudinal Reasoning Demonstrated:**

  Pattern Recognition Over Time: Jennifer identified gradual cognitive decline that might have been dismissed in episodic care

  Adaptive Goal-Setting: Targets adjusted based on TIA risk and aging

  Sustained Relationship: Trust built over 5 years enabled difficult conversations about cognition and driving

Coordinated Transitions: Maintained continuity through specialist consultations and acute event

Individualized Evidence: Applied guidelines flexibly based on patient's evolving context

- **Integration with Other Domains:**

  Acute Care: TIA required emergent response

  Preventative Care: Primary prevention (prediabetes) became secondary prevention (post-TIA)

  Interdisciplinary Care: Coordination with neurology, neuropsychology, diabetes education

  Specialty Care: Gerontologic expertise in managing multiple age-related conditions

- **Discussion Questions:**
  1. How does Jennifer's 5-year perspective differ from managing each visit in isolation?
  2. What would have been lost without sustained relationship and continuity?
  3. How did she balance evidence-based targets with patient preferences over time?
  4. When did she appropriately adjust goals based on changed circumstances?
  5. How did longitudinal accountability shape her clinical decisions?

Clinical Reflection: Longitudinal Relationships in Psychiatric Care

Working remotely in my own telehealth practice has fundamentally changed how I deliver psychiatric care—and demonstrated advantages that extend far beyond convenience.

Telehealth has dramatically improved patient access and treatment compliance. Patients can see me rapidly, without transportation barriers, childcare conflicts, or time off from work. This increased accessibility has allowed me to evaluate and treat acute psychiatric conditions that might otherwise have gone unaddressed. I've managed acute psychosis in patients who, without telehealth access, might have waited weeks for an appointment or ended up in an emergency department because outpatient care wasn't available when they needed it. Telehealth hasn't just made care more convenient—it has made care possible for patients who face structural barriers to in-person treatment.

Equally important, owning my own practice has freed me from the time constraints that fragmented my clinical work in employed settings. I'm not limited to 15-minute medication checks or pressured to see a certain number of patients per hour to meet productivity metrics. I can spend the time each patient needs—listening to their stories, understanding their concerns, exploring the context that shapes their mental health. This isn't inefficiency; it's the foundation of effective psychiatric care. The therapeutic relationship, built through sustained attention and genuine engagement, is not ancillary to treatment—it is treatment.

This longitudinal engagement has allowed me to develop deep knowledge of my patients over time. I know their baseline presentation, their patterns of decompensation, the subtle shifts in affect or thought process that signal emerging crisis. That familiarity allows me to detect changes early—before a depressive episode becomes suicidal ideation, before anxiety escalates to panic, before medication side effects prompt discontinuation. This is Chronic Care and Preventative Care functioning together: sustained relationships that enable early intervention and risk mitigation.

Suicide risk assessment, in particular, benefits from longitudinal knowledge. When I assess a patient for suicidal ideation, I'm not starting from scratch. I know their history, their prior attempts, their protective factors, their typical coping mechanisms. I can distinguish a passive wish to die from active planning. I can calibrate my response based on knowledge accumulated over months or years of treatment rather than relying solely on what they disclose in a single encounter. That depth of relationship—built through time, trust, and consistent availability—saves lives.

I'm not perfect. No clinician is. But I strive to provide the best care possible, and my patient reviews reflect that commitment. More importantly, my patients stay in treatment. They return for follow-up. They reach out when they're struggling. That continuity is the ultimate measure of effective psychiatric care—not billing codes or productivity metrics, but sustained therapeutic relationships that support recovery over time.

This is what autonomous practice makes possible: clinical decision-making aligned with patient need rather than organizational efficiency, time allocated based on clinical judgment rather than imposed schedules, and care relationships that persist because they're built on trust rather than volume. It's what nursopathic medicine describes—practicing medicine through a nursing framework that prioritizes relationship, context, and longitudinal engagement.

This experience demonstrates the Chronic Care domain in psychiatric practice. Longitudinal engagement isn't just about managing chronic illness—it's about building the depth of knowledge that enables nuanced clinical judgment. In mental health care, the therapeutic relationship is both the context for treatment and a therapeutic intervention itself. Sustained engagement over time allows me to detect subtle changes, assess risk with greater accuracy, and intervene before crises escalate. This is Chronic Care functioning as it should: continuous monitoring, evolving understanding, and trust built through consistent availability.

CHAPTER SUMMARY

Chronic Care within nursopathic medicine reflects the nurse practitioner's sustained authority and accountability for patient outcomes over time. By emphasizing continuity, adaptability, and outcome-based reasoning, this domain distinguishes autonomous practice from episodic care and reinforces the nurse practitioner's role as a consistent clinical decision-maker across the trajectory of health and illness.

CHAPTER 9
PRACTICE QUESTIONS

MULTIPLE CHOICE QUESTIONS

1. **Chronic Care is characterized by:**
   A. Single episodic encounters
   B. Sustained responsibility for monitoring and management over time
   C. Acute emergencies
   D. Preventive screening only

2. **Longitudinal clinical reasoning:**
   A. Occurs in single encounters
   B. Unfolds across repeated encounters, recognizing patterns over time
   C. Is unnecessary for experienced NPs
   D. Requires specialist consultation

3. **A defining feature of Chronic Care is:**
   A. Episodic treatment
   B. Continuous monitoring of therapeutic effectiveness and safety
   C. Crisis management
   D. Single diagnosis focus

4. **Outcome evaluation in Chronic Care extends beyond symptom control to include:**
   A. Only lab values
   B. Functional status, quality of life, and risk mitigation
   C. Patient satisfaction scores only
   D. Medication adherence alone

5. **Longitudinal accountability requires:**
   A. Seeing patients frequently
   B. Deliberate reflection on whether clinical goals are being met
   C. Specialty referral for all conditions
   D. Rigid adherence to initial treatment plans

6. **Continuity in Chronic Care is:**
   A. A passive outcome
   B. An active process requiring intentional communication and coordination
   C. Automatic
   D. Unnecessary with electronic records

7. **The therapeutic relationship in Chronic Care:**
   A. Is a barrier to objectivity
   B. Serves as both clinical insight source and foundation for shared decision-making
   C. Should be avoided
   D. Only matters in mental health

8. **As conditions evolve, initial diagnoses and management strategies:**
   A. Must never change
   B. May require revision, authority includes ability to reassess and recalibrate
   C. Should be deferred to specialists
   D. Are permanent

9. **An AGPCNP managing a patient's diabetes, hypertension, and heart failure for five years demonstrates:**
   A. Fragmented care
   B. Longitudinal reasoning, continuity, and sustained accountability
   C. Inability to refer
   D. Scope creep

10. **Chronic Care occurs:**
   A. Only in primary care
   B. Across all NP specialties regardless of setting or population
   C. Only with elderly patients
   D. Only in outpatient clinics

CASE-BASED APPLICATION QUESTIONS

Case Scenario 1:

Jennifer has managed Mrs. Davis (now 72) for five years. Started with prediabetes/hypertension, progressed to diabetes, experienced TIA, developed mild cognitive impairment, with evolving medication regimens and goal adjustments throughout.

Questions:

- How does Jennifer's 5-year perspective differ from managing each visit in isolation?
- What would have been lost without sustained relationship and continuity?
- How did longitudinal accountability shape her clinical decisions?

Case Scenario 2:

A new graduate NP says, "I don't understand why the book keeps emphasizing 'longitudinal reasoning.' I use the same clinical reasoning in every visit whether I've seen the patient once or a hundred times."

Questions:

- How would you explain what longitudinal reasoning adds beyond single-encounter reasoning?
- Provide a specific example of a clinical decision that requires longitudinal perspective.
- Why is continuity described as "an active process" rather than automatic?

TRUE/FALSE SELF-ASSESSMENT

1. ______ Chronic Care is characterized by single episodic encounters.
2. ______ Longitudinal reasoning recognizes patterns that emerge only through sustained observation.
3. ______ Continuity happens automatically with electronic medical records.
4. ______ Outcome evaluation includes functional status and quality of life, not just symptom control.
5. ______ Chronic Care occurs only in primary care settings.

See Appendix B for complete answers and rationales.

CHAPTER 10

PREVENTATIVE CARE

LEARNING OBJECTIVES

Upon completing this chapter, students will be able to:

Define the Preventative Care domain and explain its integration across all practice settings.

Describe anticipatory clinical reasoning and systematic risk identification.

Explain risk stratification processes and their role in guiding preventive interventions.

Analyze how preventive action differs from reactive treatment while remaining evidence-based.

Apply preventative reasoning to diverse specialty contexts beyond primary care.

Evaluate when prevention is appropriate versus when it becomes overscreening or overtreatment.

Integrate Preventative Care with acute management, chronic conditions, and specialty practice.

CRITICAL THINKING QUESTIONS

Anticipatory Reasoning: Provide three examples of anticipatory clinical reasoning in your specialty. How do you identify risks before they become problems? What guides your decisions about when to intervene preventively?

Beyond Primary Care: The chapter emphasizes that Preventative Care occurs across all settings, not just primary care. If you're in a specialty or acute care role, identify three ways prevention operates in your practice. How is it different from primary care prevention?

Risk Stratification: A 45-year-old patient has family history of colon cancer, hypertension, obesity, and sedentary lifestyle. Walk through your risk stratification process: What gets prioritized? Why? How do you individualize guidelines?

Iatrogenic Risk: The chapter discusses preventing "treatment-related adverse effects." Provide examples from your specialty where treatment itself creates risks requiring preventive management. How do you balance therapeutic benefit against iatrogenic risk?

Analysis: The chapter states prevention "is not treated as an adjunct to treatment, but as a core clinical responsibility requiring judgment and prioritization." Why does this framing matter? How might it change practice?

Evaluation: In value-based care and population health models, prevention is heavily emphasized. How does the nursopathic medicine framing of Preventative Care differ from population health metrics? What's gained or lost in each approach?

Integration: Map out a complex patient case showing how Preventative Care intersects with Acute Care (secondary prevention after event), Chronic Care (preventing exacerbations), Interdisciplinary Care (coordinating screening), and Specialty Care (specialty-specific prevention).

1. PURPOSE AND SCOPE

Preventative Care represents a core domain of autonomous nurse practitioner practice focused on preventing deterioration, minimizing harm, and promoting functional outcomes across the continuum of care. This domain encompasses anticipatory reasoning, risk stratification, and preventive action applied within diverse clinical contexts and specialties.

Within nursopathic medicine, Preventative Care is understood not as a discrete service line, but as a professional obligation embedded within all clinical decision-making. Risk reduction reflects the nurse practitioner's responsibility to identify foreseeable threats to health and to intervene proactively within scope and evidence-based standards. The anticipatory reasoning method described in Chapter 4 establishes the cognitive foundation for this domain; Chapter 4 should be revisited as the conceptual anchor from which the Preventative Care domain draws its reasoning structure.

2. ANTICIPATORY CLINICAL REASONING

Preventative Care relies on anticipatory clinical reasoning, the capacity to recognize emerging risks before they manifest as acute or irreversible conditions (Tanner, 2006). Nurse practitioners apply this reasoning by integrating patient history, population-based risk factors, treatment exposures, and contextual variables to anticipate future harm.

This forward-looking approach complements acute and chronic reasoning. Rather than responding to instability or progression alone, the nurse practitioner actively works to alter trajectories through early identification and intervention.

3. RISK IDENTIFICATION AND STRATIFICATION

A defining feature of this domain is systematic risk identification. Nurse practitioners assess biological, psychological, social, and treatment-related risks that may compromise patient outcomes over time. These risks may be intrinsic to the patient, related to disease processes, or iatrogenic in nature.

Risk stratification guides the intensity and timing of preventive actions. Within the nursopathic framework, the authority to manage risk includes responsibility for selecting appropriate preventive strategies and reassessing risk as conditions evolve.

4. PREVENTIVE ACTION AND HARM MITIGATION

Preventive action within this domain encompasses screening, counseling, anticipatory guidance, and interventions designed to reduce morbidity and prevent avoidable complications. These actions are selected based on evidence, patient context, and clinical judgment rather than rote protocol adherence.

Harm mitigation extends to the prevention of treatment-related adverse effects. Nurse practitioners practicing autonomously must balance therapeutic benefit with potential risk, adjusting management strategies to preserve safety and function.

5. INTEGRATION ACROSS THE CONTINUUM OF CARE

Preventative Care is not confined to primary care or wellness settings. It occurs across acute, chronic, specialty, and procedural environments. Nurse practitioners integrate preventive reasoning into all phases of care, including during episodes of instability, recovery, and long-term management.

Within nursopathic medicine, this integration reinforces the continuity of professional responsibility. Risk reduction is not deferred or delegated, but incorporated into autonomous decision-making wherever patient vulnerability exists.

6. INTEGRATION WITH OTHER DOMAINS

Preventative Care intersects with Acute Care through secondary prevention after acute events, with Chronic Care through ongoing risk reduction in chronic conditions, with Interdisciplinary Care when coordinating preventive strategies with other providers, and with Specialty Care when applying population-specific prevention guidelines.

7. DURABILITY ACROSS SETTINGS AND SPECIALTIES

The durability of this domain lies in its universality. All nurse practitioner specialties encounter preventable risk and possess the authority to intervene within scope. By framing prevention as a function of clinical reasoning rather than a checklist of services, this domain remains applicable across populations, practice settings, and evolving standards of care.

8. ILLUSTRATIVE EXAMPLES ACROSS SPECIALTIES

- **Family NP:** Evidence-guided screening and counseling to reduce long-term disease risk, including cardiovascular risk assessment, cancer screening, and immunization administration.
- **Psychiatric-Mental Health NP:** Monitoring and mitigation of medication-related metabolic risks, suicide prevention strategies, and relapse prevention planning.
- **Adult-Gerontology NP:** Fall prevention, osteoporosis screening, polypharmacy reduction, and functional risk reduction in older adults.
- **Pediatric NP:** Developmental risk assessment, anticipatory guidance for injury prevention, and age-appropriate immunization planning.
- **Neonatal NP:** Prevention of morbidity associated with prematurity or critical illness, including infection control and developmental care strategies.
- **Emergency NP:** Secondary prevention and injury risk mitigation following acute events, such as fall prevention counseling after trauma or stroke risk assessment after TIA.

9. CASE STUDIES

Case 1: Preventative Care Across Multiple Risk Domains

- **Case Presentation:**

  Marcus Thompson, FNP, sees Mr. Robert Chen, age 52, for an annual wellness visit. This visit demonstrates how Preventative Care operates as anticipatory reasoning across multiple risk domains.

- **Initial Risk Assessment:**

  Demographics & History: Asian American male, office worker, sedentary

  Family history: Father died of MI at age 58, mother has type 2 diabetes

Social: Married, two teenagers, high-stress job (recent promotion to management)

Habits: Non-smoker, 2-3 alcoholic drinks nightly, no regular exercise

Sleep: 5-6 hours nightly, snores loudly (per wife), daytime fatigue

Current Health:

BP: 138/88 (repeated: 142/90)

BMI: 29.5 (overweight, approaching obese)

Labs: HbA1c 5.8%, LDL 142, HDL 38, TG 180

Screening questionnaires: PHQ-9 score 8 (mild depression), GAD-7 score 11 (moderate anxiety)

- **Marcus's Anticipatory Clinical Reasoning:**

  Rather than simply treating each finding in isolation, Marcus conducts comprehensive risk stratification across multiple domains:

- **Cardiovascular Risk (Primary Prevention - High Priority):**

  10-year ASCVD risk: 12.8% (elevated for age)

  Multiple risk factors clustering: prehypertension, prediabetes, dyslipidemia, family history, stress, sedentary lifestyle

  Prevention Plan:

  - Initiates moderate-intensity statin (atorvastatin 20 mg)
  - Sets BP target <130/80 given diabetes risk
  - Recommends cardiac calcium scoring if patient wants more data
  - Shared decision-making about aspirin (decided against given low-dose aspirin trial data)

- **Metabolic Risk (Diabetes Prevention - High Priority):**

  Prediabetes with strong family history and multiple risk factors

  Prevention Plan:

  - Refers to Diabetes Prevention Program (lifestyle intervention)

    - Discusses metformin for prevention (patient prefers lifestyle first)
    - Schedules 3-month follow-up for HbA1c recheck rather than annual
    - Goal: prevent or delay progression to diabetes
- **Sleep Apnea Risk (Often Overlooked - Medium Priority):**

  Classic presentation: overweight, loud snoring, daytime fatigue, hypertension

  Untreated OSA increases cardiovascular and metabolic risk

  Prevention Plan:

    - Orders home sleep apnea test
    - Educates about OSA cardiovascular impact
    - Plans CPAP initiation if positive (which would also help BP and fatigue)
- **Mental Health Risk (Integrated Prevention - Medium Priority):**

  Mild depression and moderate anxiety in context of job stress

  Risk for progression, impact on medication adherence, cardiovascular effects of chronic stress

  Prevention Plan:

    - Recommends stress management/mindfulness program
    - Provides resources for therapy (patient interested)
    - Monitors, will consider SSRI if worsens or lifestyle changes insufficient
    - Notes anxiety/depression can sabotage other preventive efforts
- **Fall/Injury Risk (Lower Priority Now, But Establishing Baseline):**

  Currently low risk, but establishing exercise habit now prevents future frailty

  Prevention Plan:

  - Emphasizes weight-bearing exercise for cardiovascular AND future bone health
  - Establishes baseline for functional status

- **Cancer Screening (Age-Appropriate):**

  Due for colorectal cancer screening (age 52, family history)

  Prevention Plan:

  - Orders FIT testing (patient prefers over colonoscopy initially)
  - Schedules colonoscopy for following year if family history warrants

- **Anticipatory Guidance - Future Risks:**

  Marcus discusses:

  - Alcohol use (trending toward problematic, moderate consumption recommended)
  - Work-life balance (burnout prevention)
  - Sleep hygiene (independent of apnea treatment)
  - Injury prevention (ergonomics for office work)

- **Integration with Other Domains:**

  Acute Care: If Mr. Chen had chest pain today, his risk profile would inform urgency

  Chronic Care: If prevention fails and diabetes develops, transition to chronic management

  Interdisciplinary Care: Referrals to DPP, sleep medicine, mental health

  Specialty Care: Uses knowledge of cardiovascular and metabolic prevention strategies

- **Three-Month Follow-Up:**

  Mr. Chen returns:

  - Started DPP, lost 8 pounds
  - Sleep study positive for moderate OSA, started CPAP (tolerating well)
  - BP now 128/82 (off medication, improved with weight loss and CPAP!)

    - Reports feeling "more energetic," started walking during lunch breaks
    - HbA1c: 5.6% (improved)
    - Seeing therapist, anxiety better managed

- **Outcome:**

  Marcus's comprehensive risk stratification and anticipatory reasoning potentially prevented:

    - Myocardial infarction (father's age at death: 58; Mr. Chen is 52)
    - Type 2 diabetes progression
    - Cardiovascular complications from untreated OSA
    - Mental health deterioration affecting overall health

  His approach demonstrates prevention as active clinical reasoning, not passive screening checkboxes.

- **Discussion Questions:**

  1. How did Marcus prioritize among multiple competing risks?
  2. What role did patient engagement and shared decision-making play?
  3. How might this approach differ from protocol-driven prevention?
  4. What was gained by integrating mental health into cardiovascular/metabolic prevention?
  5. How does anticipatory reasoning differ from reactive treatment?
  6. What evidence guided each preventive intervention?

CHAPTER SUMMARY

Preventative Care within nursopathic medicine reflects the nurse practitioner's proactive responsibility to prevent harm and promote sustainable outcomes. By emphasizing anticipatory reasoning, systematic risk assessment, and preventive action, this domain reinforces autonomy as an ongoing obligation rather than a reactive role, applicable across all specialties and care settings.

CHAPTER 10
PRACTICE QUESTIONS

MULTIPLE CHOICE QUESTIONS

1. **Preventative Care in nursopathic medicine is:**
   A. A discrete service line
   B. A professional obligation embedded within all clinical decision-making
   C. Only performed in wellness visits
   D. The same as public health

2. **Anticipatory clinical reasoning involves:**
   A. Reactive treatment
   B. Recognizing emerging risks before they manifest as acute conditions
   C. Crisis management
   D. Specialist referral

3. **Risk stratification in Preventative Care guides:**
   A. Billing codes
   B. The intensity and timing of preventive actions
   C. Medication costs
   D. Appointment scheduling

4. **Prevention in nursopathic medicine includes all EXCEPT:**
   A. Screening
   B. Anticipatory guidance
   C. Waiting for symptoms to appear
   D. Harm mitigation

5. **Harm mitigation extends to prevention of:**
   A. Legal liability only
   B. Treatment-related adverse effects
   C. Patient complaints
   D. Regulatory violations

6. **Preventative Care occurs:**
   A. Only in primary care settings
   B. Across acute, chronic, specialty, and procedural environments
   C. Only during wellness visits
   D. Only with healthy patients

7. **A PMHNP monitoring metabolic risks from antipsychotic medications demonstrates:**
   A. Acute Care
   B. Preventative Care, anticipatory harm mitigation
   C. Chronic Care only
   D. Overstepping scope

8. **The chapter states prevention is:**
   A. An adjunct to treatment
   B. Not treated as adjunct but as core clinical responsibility
   C. Optional based on time
   D. Only for healthy patients

9. **Anticipatory guidance differs from reactive treatment by:**
   A. Being less important
   B. Identifying and addressing risks before problems occur
   C. Requiring specialist training
   D. Being impossible to document

10. An AGACNP implementing fall prevention strategies in a hospitalized elder is performing:

A. Outside NP scope

B. Preventative Care integrated into acute care setting

C. Only nursing assistant tasks

D. Physical therapy

CASE-BASED APPLICATION QUESTIONS

Case Scenario 1:

Marcus sees Mr. Chen, 52, for annual wellness. Multiple clustering risk factors: prehypertension, prediabetes, dyslipidemia, family history of MI at 58, stress, sedentary lifestyle, possible sleep apnea, mild depression/anxiety.

Questions:

- How does Marcus's comprehensive risk stratification differ from addressing each finding in isolation?
- Explain how prevention operates across multiple risk domains simultaneously.
- Why is this approach described as "anticipatory reasoning" rather than "screening"?

Case Scenario 2:

A student asks, "Isn't prevention just following guidelines, like checking the USPSTF recommendations and ordering the tests? Why does it require 'clinical judgment'?"

Questions:

- How would you explain that prevention requires judgment beyond guideline implementation?
- Give an example where guidelines must be individualized based on patient context.

- Why is prevention considered a "core clinical responsibility" rather than task completion?

TRUE/FALSE SELF-ASSESSMENT

1. ______ Preventative Care is a discrete service line separate from other domains.
2. ______ Anticipatory reasoning identifies risks before they become acute conditions.
3. ______ Preventative Care occurs only during wellness visits.
4. ______ A PMHNP monitoring metabolic effects of antipsychotics is practicing Preventative Care.
5. ______ Preventive actions follow protocols rigidly without clinical judgment.

See Appendix B for complete answers and rationales.

CHAPTER 11

INTERDISCIPLINARY CARE

LEARNING OBJECTIVES

Upon completing this chapter, students will be able to:

Define the Interdisciplinary Care domain and explain its role in autonomous practice.

Distinguish collaboration from dependency in professional relationships.

Describe the interdisciplinary interface where expertise is exchanged without transferring accountability.

Identify key interdisciplinary relationships for NPs (MDs/DOs, PharmDs, DPTs, PsyDs, ODs, DPMs, DDS/DMDs, DCs).

Explain how to maintain autonomous authority while engaging in meaningful collaboration.

Analyze when consultation, referral, co-management, or coordination is clinically appropriate.

Apply ethical principles of collaboration including recognition of limits and professional respect.

CRITICAL THINKING QUESTIONS

The Vine Metaphor: Recall the green vine from Chapter 7 symbolizing collaboration that's "too tight constricts, too loose fumbles." Provide clinical examples of each extreme and describe what balanced collaboration looks like in your specialty.

Collaboration vs. Dependency: You're required to have a "collaborative agreement" with a physician as a regulatory requirement, but your state law grants you independent prescriptive authority. How do you maintain autonomous practice (collaboration without dependency) in this situation?

Interdisciplinary Interface: Map out a complex patient case requiring multiple disciplines. At each interface (NP-MD, NP-PharmD, NP-PT, etc.), identify: What expertise is being exchanged? Who retains what accountability? How is coordination maintained?

Professional Respect: You consult a specialist who responds condescendingly, suggesting you should "let real doctors handle" complex cases. Using this chapter's framework, how do you respond in a way that maintains professionalism while asserting your autonomous authority?

Recognition of Limits: Describe a situation where recognizing the limits of your expertise and consulting/referring is not a limitation of autonomy but an expression of professional responsibility. How do you determine when consultation is needed?

Evaluation: Some healthcare systems emphasize "team-based care" where all decisions are made collectively. How does this approach align or conflict with the Interdisciplinary Care domain as described? Can autonomous practice exist in highly collaborative environments?

Synthesis: Design an interdisciplinary practice model for a specific clinical context (primary care clinic, hospital unit, specialty practice, etc.). How would you structure roles, decision-making, communication, and accountability to achieve the balance the vine metaphor represents?

1. PURPOSE AND SCOPE

Interdisciplinary Care represents a fundamental domain of autonomous nurse practitioner practice that acknowledges modern healthcare as inherently collaborative, requiring coordination to optimize outcomes, and patient experience (Interprofessional Education Collaborative, 2016; World Health Organization, 2010). This domain describes how nurse practitioners engage with professionals across multiple disciplines to enhance patient outcomes while maintaining independent clinical authority and accountability within nursing scope.

Within nursopathic medicine, Interdisciplinary Care is neither subordination nor isolation. It is the purposeful integration of diverse expertise through clearly defined professional relationships that respect autonomy, clarify responsibility, and prioritize patient benefit.

2. THE NATURE OF INTERDISCIPLINARY COLLABORATION

Contemporary healthcare requires coordination across multiple disciplines, each contributing specialized knowledge to comprehensive patient care. Nurse practitioners routinely engage with allopathic and osteopathic physicians, pharmacists, physical therapists, psychologists, dentists, optometrists, podiatrists, chiropractors, and other licensed professionals.

Effective interdisciplinary practice depends on role clarity. When each discipline's scope, authority, and accountability are well-defined, collaboration becomes a mechanism for integrating expertise rather than negotiating hierarchy. Nurse practitioners contribute autonomous clinical judgment while benefiting from the specialized knowledge of other professionals.

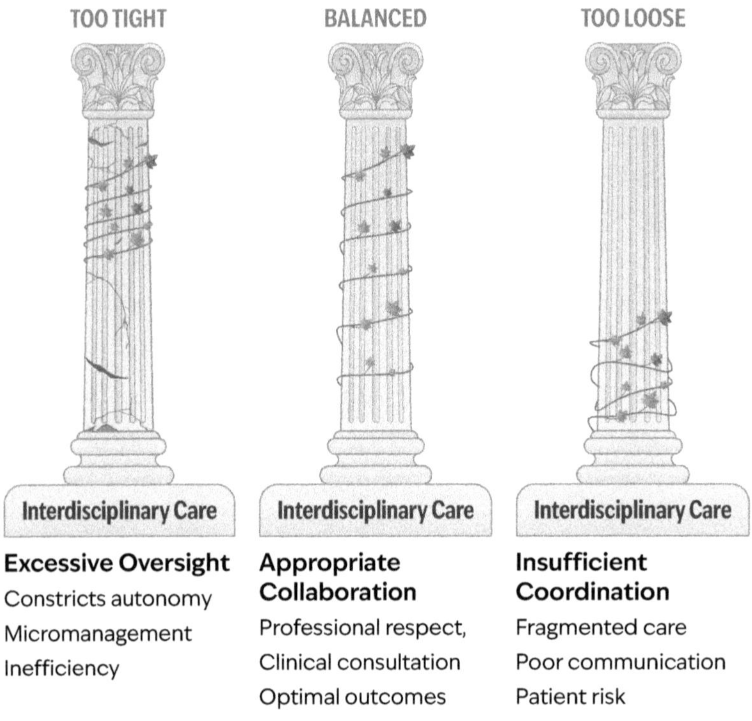

Figure 11.1. Finding Balance in Interdisciplinary Collaboration.

3. COLLABORATION DISTINGUISHED FROM DEPENDENCY

A critical feature of this domain is the distinction between collaboration and dependency. Collaboration occurs when professionals engage as equals, each exercising independent judgment within their respective scopes, rather than subordination or hierarchy (World Health Organization, 2010). Dependency occurs when one professional's authority is contingent upon another's approval or oversight regardless of clinical necessity.

Within nursopathic medicine, Interdisciplinary Care is collaborative. Nurse practitioners consult, refer, and coordinate with other disciplines based on clinical indication, not regulatory requirement. This approach preserves accountability by ensuring that the clinician responsible for patient outcomes retains decision-making authority. The interdisciplinary reasoning method articulated in Chapter 4 provides the conceptual framework that makes this domain coherent; readers are encouraged to revisit Chapter 4's treatment of interdisciplinary reasoning as the methodological foundation for the domain developed here.

4. THE INTERDISCIPLINARY INTERFACE

Interdisciplinary Care functions most effectively at clearly defined interfaces where expertise is exchanged without transferring accountability (IPEC, 2016; Hamric et al., 2014). These interfaces occur through:

- **Consultation:** Seeking expert opinion while retaining primary responsibility for clinical decisions and management.
- **Referral:** Transferring specific aspects of care to another professional whose expertise is required, while maintaining overall care coordination.
- **Co-management:** Sharing ongoing responsibility for specific clinical problems, with clear delineation of each discipline's role.
- **Coordination:** Integrating multiple providers' contributions into a coherent care plan under the nurse practitioner's autonomous management.

At each interface, professional boundaries remain clear, reducing ambiguity and supporting patient safety.

5. KEY INTERDISCIPLINARY RELATIONSHIPS

Nurse practitioners engage with diverse healthcare disciplines, each relationship characterized by mutual respect and defined scope:

- **Allopathic and Osteopathic Medicine (MD/DO):** Collaboration with physicians across specialties for consultation on complex cases, specialty referrals, or co-management of conditions requiring multidisciplinary expertise. Nurse practitioners maintain autonomous primary care or specialty management while accessing physician expertise when indicated.

- **Pharmacy (PharmD):** Collaborative medication management, including pharmacist consultation on complex regimens, drug interactions, or specialty medications. Nurse practitioners retain prescriptive authority while benefiting from pharmacologic expertise.
- **Physical Therapy (DPT):** Referral and coordination for rehabilitation, functional restoration, and mobility optimization. Nurse practitioners integrate physical therapy recommendations into complete care plans.
- **Psychology (PsyD):** Collaboration in mental health care, including referral for psychotherapy, psychological testing, or behavioral interventions. Psychiatric-mental health nurse practitioners may co-manage patients receiving both psychopharmacologic and psychotherapeutic treatment.
- **Optometry (OD):** Referral for comprehensive eye examinations, vision correction, and ocular disease management. Nurse practitioners coordinate care when systemic conditions affect ocular health.
- **Podiatric Medicine (DPM):** Consultation and referral for foot and ankle conditions, particularly in patients with diabetes or vascular disease requiring specialized podiatric intervention.
- **Dentistry (DDS/DMD):** Coordination of oral health with systemic health, particularly in patients with conditions affecting or affected by dental health.
- **Chiropractic Medicine (DC):** Referral for musculoskeletal conditions when chiropractic intervention is appropriate, with ongoing coordination of pain management and functional outcomes.

6. MAINTAINING AUTONOMY WITHIN INTERDISCIPLINARY SYSTEMS

Autonomous practice within interdisciplinary environments requires clarity about when collaboration enhances care versus when it creates unnecessary dependency. Nurse practitioners exercise judgment in determining when:

- **Independent management** is appropriate and within scope
- **Consultation** would enhance clinical decision-making
- **Referral** is necessary due to complexity or specialty expertise requirements
- **Co-management** optimizes outcomes through shared responsibility

This judgment is grounded in clinical competence, scope awareness, and commitment to patient safety rather than hierarchical models or professional deference.

7. COMMUNICATION AND PROFESSIONAL RESPECT

Effective Interdisciplinary Care requires clear, timely, and respectful communication. Nurse practitioners engage other professionals as colleagues, clearly articulating clinical questions, sharing relevant information, and integrating recommendations into autonomous decision-making.

Professional respect is bidirectional. Nurse practitioners expect their autonomous authority to be recognized just as they recognize the expertise and authority of other disciplines. This mutual respect supports functional collaboration without role confusion.

8. INTEGRATION WITH OTHER DOMAINS

Interdisciplinary Care permeates all other domains of nursopathic medicine:

- **Acute Care:** Consultation with specialists during acute crises or emergency situations

- **Chronic Care:** Coordination with multiple providers managing different aspects of chronic conditions
- **Preventative Care:** Referral to specialists for screening procedures or risk-specific interventions
- **Specialty Care:** Collaboration with physicians and other specialists practicing in related fields

Rather than functioning in isolation, Interdisciplinary Care operates as an overlay across the full scope of autonomous practice.

9. ETHICAL DIMENSIONS OF COLLABORATION

Interdisciplinary collaboration carries ethical obligations. Nurse practitioners must:

- Recognize the limits of their expertise and consult appropriately
- Ensure continuity and coordination to prevent fragmented care
- Maintain clear accountability even when multiple providers are involved
- Prioritize patient benefit over professional territoriality
- Communicate transparently with patients about who is responsible for their care

These ethical commitments reinforce that autonomy includes the responsibility to engage others when patient welfare requires it.

10. DURABILITY ACROSS SETTINGS

Interdisciplinary Care occurs in every practice environment. Whether in primary care clinics, hospitals, psychiatric facilities, specialty practices, or community settings, nurse practitioners navigate complex professional relationships. The durability of this domain reflects the reality that healthcare is fundamentally collaborative, requiring clear professional identity within team-based systems.

Clinical Reflection: Navigating Interdisciplinary Collaboration in Evolving Professional Boundaries

Working in my own practice has taught me that autonomous practice is both rewarding and demanding. You are constantly managing not just clinical care, but the operational, regulatory, and interprofessional challenges that come with independent decision-making. One area where I've continually learned and grown is effective interdisciplinary collaboration, particularly with pharmacists.

I've had the privilege of collaborating with exceptional colleagues—including Dr. Monica Barfield, DNP, APRN, and other independent nurse practitioners—in the shared care of mutual patients. These collaborations have been productive and have reinforced my belief that interdisciplinary care enhances rather than replaces autonomous practice. When done well, collaboration means consulting as professional peers, sharing clinical reasoning, and coordinating care while each practitioner maintains independent judgment within their scope.

My relationship with pharmacists has been similarly collaborative in many respects. Pharmacists serve an essential role in medication safety, and their clinical expertise has genuinely improved my prescribing on multiple occasions. They catch potential drug interactions I might have missed, alert me to dosing concerns based on patient-specific factors, and provide valuable input on medication alternatives when insurance formularies or patient tolerability become issues. This professional consultation is exactly what interdisciplinary care should look like—each profession contributing unique expertise to enhance patient outcomes.

However, as a psychiatric-mental health nurse practitioner prescribing controlled substances in a telehealth practice, I've also navigated the complexity of evolving professional boundaries. Pharmacists, like all healthcare professionals, were trained in models where nurse practitioner prescribing authority was more limited than current state regulations allow. When those historical models inform current practice patterns, questions sometimes arise about prescribing authority that reflect genuine uncertainty about what nurse practitioners can prescribe rather than intentional resistance to NP autonomy.

The regulatory landscape contributes to this complexity in ways that affect all prescribers. Pharmacy rules and regulations vary significantly—not just between states, but sometimes between individual pharmacies or pharmacy chains based on internal policies, corporate risk management decisions, or differences in how regulations are interpreted. What one pharmacy dispenses routinely, another may question, creating inconsistency that affects patient access to necessary medications. This is particularly challenging in mental health care, where continuity and consistency of treatment are essential for therapeutic effectiveness.

As of this writing, the DEA has not yet finalized regulations on telehealth prescribing of controlled substances, creating significant uncertainty for all telehealth prescribers—physicians, nurse practitioners, and physician assistants alike. This regulatory ambiguity creates challenges for pharmacists as well, who must balance patient access needs against uncertain regulatory guidance and potential liability concerns. The challenge isn't that pharmacists are creating barriers—it's that the regulatory environment hasn't caught up with how healthcare is actually being delivered, leaving everyone navigating uncertain terrain.

In my practice, I take additional steps to ensure appropriate controlled substance prescribing, including obtaining urine drug confirmation panels to verify patient compliance, maintaining detailed documentation of clinical rationale, and consulting evidence-based guidelines for psychiatric pharmacotherapy. I do this not because it's legally required, but because controlled substance prescribing carries significant responsibility, and thorough documentation supports both patient safety and professional accountability. When pharmacists request additional information, I view it as an opportunity to demonstrate that NP prescribing is grounded in the same rigorous clinical reasoning and safety protocols that guide physician prescribing.

What this experience has taught me is that interdisciplinary collaboration in healthcare requires ongoing adaptation as professional scopes evolve. Pharmacists are navigating the same changing landscape that nurse practitioners are—trying to understand expanded scopes, uncertain regulations, and evolving professional boundaries while maintaining their essential role in medication safety. The solution isn't to view questions or requests for documentation as obstacles, but to recognize them as part of a healthcare system adapting to change. Clear frameworks—like nursopathic medicine—that explain how nurse practitioners exercise independent clinical authority help all healthcare professionals understand how to collaborate effectively.

This experience illustrates both the value and complexity of interdisciplinary collaboration when professional scopes are evolving. Pharmacists provide essential medication safety expertise that genuinely improves patient care. Their questions about prescribing authority often reflect the healthcare system's ongoing adaptation to expanded nurse practitioner scope rather than resistance to NP autonomy. True collaboration requires mutual respect for each profession's independent scope and judgment—and mutual understanding that we're all navigating regulatory uncertainty and changing professional boundaries together.

The framework of nursopathic medicine helps address this challenge by providing conceptual clarity about how nurse practitioners exercise autonomous clinical authority. When all healthcare professionals understand that NPs practice medicine through a distinct nursing framework with independent diagnostic and therapeutic authority grounded in graduate education and state licensure, collaboration becomes easier. Pharmacists can engage with NP prescribers as autonomous professionals while maintaining their essential medication safety role. The vine of collaboration supports the structure when it's calibrated appropriately—neither so tight that it constricts professional autonomy, nor so loose that it abandons the collaborative partnerships that enhance patient care.

CHAPTER SUMMARY

Interdisciplinary Care within nursopathic medicine represents the nurse practitioner's engagement with multiple healthcare disciplines to enhance patient outcomes while maintaining autonomous clinical authority. This domain is characterized by purposeful collaboration, clear professional boundaries, and mutual respect. Effective interdisciplinary practice requires distinguishing collaboration from dependency, maintaining accountability, and prioritizing patient benefit. By defining how nurse practitioners work with other professions, this domain affirms that autonomy and teamwork are complementary rather than oppositional.

CHAPTER 11
PRACTICE QUESTIONS

MULTIPLE CHOICE QUESTIONS

1. **Interdisciplinary Care is defined as:**
   A. Required supervision by physicians
   B. Collaborative engagement across professions while maintaining autonomous clinical authority
   C. Replacing autonomous decision-making
   D. Delegation of responsibilities

2. **The green vine metaphor represents:**
   A. Organic nursing practice
   B. Unity in collaboration, balanced to neither constrict nor fumble care
   C. Natural healing processes
   D. Hospital hierarchies

3. **When the vine is "too tight," it symbolizes:**
   A. Good structure and support
   B. Excessive oversight that constricts care and limits autonomous judgment
   C. Appropriate collaboration
   D. Patient safety

4. **When the vine is "too loose," it symbolizes:**
   A. Maximum autonomy
   B. Care fumbled through insufficient coordination and fragmented delivery
   C. Independence
   D. Reduced liability

5. **Interdisciplinary collaboration in nursopathic medicine:**
   A. Replaces autonomous practice
   B. Operates alongside autonomous practice
   C. Is only required by regulation
   D. Indicates incompetence

6. **The NP's role in interdisciplinary teams involves:**
   A. Subordination to physicians
   B. Autonomous clinical contribution within nursing's professional framework
   C. Task delegation only
   D. No independent decision-making

7. **Consultation differs from supervision in that consultation:**
   A. Is mandatory by regulation
   B. Is chosen based on clinical need, not hierarchical requirement
   C. Indicates lack of competence
   D. Transfers accountability

8. **Appropriate interdisciplinary engagement requires:**
   A. Physician approval for all decisions
   B. Clear communication while maintaining professional accountability
   C. Abandoning autonomous judgment
   D. Avoiding collaboration

9. **The balance metaphor (vine neither too tight nor too loose) teaches that:**
   A. Collaboration is unnecessary
   B. Professional relationships require thoughtful calibration
   C. More oversight is always better
   D. Independence means isolation

10. **An NP consulting cardiology for a complex patient demonstrates:**
    A. Inability to practice independently
    B. Professional maturity recognizing when specialist input enhances care
    C. Scope violation
    D. Regulatory compliance only

CASE-BASED APPLICATION QUESTIONS

Case Scenario 1:

In one hospital, AGACNPs must obtain physician co-signature on all orders before implementation, even for routine care within established protocols. In another hospital, AGACNPs round independently, consult specialists based on clinical judgment, and collaborate as professional peers.

Questions:

- Using the vine metaphor, how would you characterize these two models?;
- What are the consequences of each model for patient care and professional practice?
- How does the second model demonstrate the Interdisciplinary Care domain?

Case Scenario 2:

Sarah, a PMHNP, is managing a complex patient with treatment-resistant depression and new cardiac symptoms. She consults cardiology, who recommends a medication adjustment that could interact with psychiatric medications. Sarah discusses the interaction concerns and they collaborate to find a solution safe for both conditions.

Questions:

- How does this scenario demonstrate autonomous practice coexisting with collaboration?
- Why is this interdisciplinary engagement, not supervision?
- What would "vine too tight" or "vine too loose" look like in this scenario?

TRUE/FALSE SELF-ASSESSMENT

1. ______ Interdisciplinary Care replaces autonomous decision-making.
2. ______ The vine metaphor teaches that collaboration requires thoughtful balance.
3. ______ When the vine is "too tight," it provides appropriate structure and support.
4. ______ Consultation based on clinical judgment demonstrates professional maturity, not incompetence.
5. ______ Interdisciplinary engagement transfers accountability from the NP to consultants.

See Appendix B for complete answers and rationales.

CHAPTER 12

SPECIALTY CARE

LEARNING OBJECTIVES

Upon completing this chapter, students will be able to:

Define the Specialty Care domain and explain how specialization refines autonomous practice.

Distinguish between employment setting and practice scope, including certification requirements.

Explain nursing's distinct approach to specialty practice (population/context-focused vs. organ-system focused).

Analyze when specialty practice is appropriate based on education, certification, and competency.

Describe how emerging specialty roles (oncology NP, cardiology NP, etc.) fit within nursopathic medicine.

Evaluate scope boundaries and the principle that authority must match competency.

Apply principles of consultation and recognition of limits in specialty practice.

CRITICAL THINKING QUESTIONS

Scope Alignment: An FNP is offered a position in an orthopedic surgery practice managing pre- and post-operative patients. Using this chapter's framework, what questions must be addressed before accepting? What would constitute appropriate versus inappropriate practice?

Nursing's Approach: Compare how a cardiologist and a cardiology-certified NP might approach the same heart failure patient. What's similar? What makes the NP's approach distinctly nursing-centered despite managing the same condition?

Emerging Roles: Research an emerging NP specialty role (dermoscopy, GI, interventional, etc.). How does it fit within the nursopathic framework? What education/certification supports autonomous practice in this area?

Analysis: The chapter discusses Peplau's psychiatric nurses "applying psychological knowledge through a nursing framework" as precedent for specialty NPs applying specialty medical knowledge through nursing. Explain this parallel and evaluate whether it's convincing.

Ethical Scenario: You're an FNP working in a cardiology clinic. The cardiologist is on vacation and a patient calls with new severe chest pain. Your scope includes managing stable chronic heart disease, but this is an acute, complex presentation. Walk through your decision-making using this chapter's principles about scope, competency, and limits.

Certification vs. Experience: Some argue that extensive experience in a specialty setting is equivalent to formal certification. Using this chapter, construct an argument for why formal education and certification matter even with experience. Then construct the counter-argument. Which is more compelling?

Synthesis: Design an educational pathway for NPs wanting to develop subspecialty expertise. What combination of didactic education, clinical experience, certification, and mentorship would appropriately prepare someone for autonomous specialty practice?

1. PURPOSE AND SCOPE

Specialty Care represents the domain in which nurse practitioner expertise is refined to address the unique needs of defined populations, conditions, or clinical contexts (Kleinpell et al., 2014; Hamric et al., 2014). This domain acknowledges that while the functions of autonomous practice remain constant, their expression is shaped by specialized knowledge, skills, and clinical focus.

Within nursopathic medicine, specialization does not fragment professional identity or authority. Instead, it sharpens clinical reasoning, allowing nurse practitioners to apply the same foundational domains (Acute Care, Chronic Care, Preventative Care, and Interdisciplinary Care) through a focused clinical lens.

2. SCOPE ALIGNMENT AND CERTIFICATION REQUIREMENTS

Specialty Care within nursopathic medicine requires rigorous alignment between education, certification, licensure, and clinical practice (APRN Joint Dialogue Group, 2008; National Council of State Boards of Nursing, 2008). Autonomous practice is exercised within the specialty for which the nurse practitioner is formally educated and nationally certified, not simply the setting in which they are employed. The specialty lens reasoning method described in Chapter 4 establishes the cognitive architecture underlying this domain; that chapter provides the foundational framework that explains how a specialty lens filters clinical information differently from a generalist lens while remaining grounded in the same nursing identity.

3. EDUCATION AND CERTIFICATION AS PREREQUISITES

Graduate nursing education prepares nurse practitioners for specific population foci and practice contexts (NCSBN, 2008; AACN, 2021). National certification verifies specialty competency through validated assessment in the area in which the NP is expected to practice (National Organization of Nurse Practitioner Faculties, 2017). Autonomous specialty practice requires:

- **Graduate-level education** in the specialty area, whether through initial NP preparation or formal post-graduate fellowship/certificate programs

- **National certification** in the specialty when available (e.g., family, adult-gerontology primary care, adult-gerontology acute care, psychiatric-mental health, neonatal, pediatric, women's health)
- **Additional specialty certification** for subspecialty practice when appropriate certifying bodies exist (e.g., oncology certification, emergency certification, dermatology certification)
- **Documented clinical competency** through supervised practice, preceptorship, or fellowship training
- **Ongoing practice** within the boundaries of one's certification and demonstrated competency

4. THE DISTINCTION BETWEEN EMPLOYMENT SETTING AND PRACTICE SCOPE

Employment in a specialty clinical setting does not, by itself, expand a nurse practitioner's scope of practice or autonomous authority. A family nurse practitioner employed in a cardiology clinic practices as a family nurse practitioner (applying FNP scope to patients within that setting) not as a cardiology specialist.

This distinction is critical for several reasons:

- **Professional Accountability:** Nurse practitioners remain accountable to their certification and licensure scope regardless of employment. Practicing beyond one's certified scope creates professional, legal, and ethical liability.
- **Patient Safety:** Specialty medical practice often involves complex pathophysiology, advanced diagnostics, and high-risk interventions that require specialized education and training. Patient safety depends on practitioners recognizing the boundaries of their competence.
- **Professional Integrity:** Nursopathic medicine is grounded in nursing's epistemology and values, not in replicating physician training pathways. Nurse practitioners do not become cardiologists, oncologists, or urologists by working in those settings. They bring nursing expertise to those populations.

- **Regulatory Clarity:** State practice acts and certification bodies define scope by population focus and practice setting (primary care, acute care, etc.), not by medical subspecialty. Practicing beyond one's defined scope, even if employed in a specialty setting, may violate regulatory standards.

5. WHEN SPECIALTY PRACTICE IS APPROPRIATE

Legitimate specialty practice within nursopathic medicine occurs when:

- **Formal education exists:** The nurse practitioner has completed graduate-level education specifically designed for that specialty (e.g., neonatal NP programs, psychiatric-mental health NP programs, acute care NP programs with specialty focus).
- **Certification is obtained:** The practitioner holds national certification validating specialty competency. Where specialty certification exists (oncology, dermatology, emergency, etc.), it should be obtained before independent specialty practice.
- **Supervised transition occurs:** Before autonomous practice, the nurse practitioner completes supervised clinical experience with specialty-specific preceptors who validate competency.
- **Scope remains clear:** The practitioner practices within nursing scope, applying advanced nursing judgment to specialty populations. Not attempting to replicate physician subspecialty training or assuming physician scope.

6. NURSING'S DISTINCT APPROACH TO SPECIALTY PRACTICE

Nursopathic medicine does not seek to replicate the physician subspecialty model. Physician subspecialties (cardiology, oncology, urology, etc.) are organized around organ systems and disease categories, requiring years of residency and fellowship training within the medical education framework.

Nurse practitioner specialty practice is organized differently:

- **Population-focused** rather than organ-system focused (adult-gerontology, pediatric, neonatal, women's health)
- **Context-focused** rather than disease-focused (primary care, acute care, psychiatric-mental health)
- **Nursing-centered** in its approach to assessment, diagnosis, and management

Grounded in nursing values of whole-person care, patient advocacy, and functional outcomes

When nurse practitioners develop subspecialty expertise (oncology, cardiology, orthopedics, etc.), they do so **as nurse practitioners**, bringing nursing's orientation to care into that specialty area. They are not junior physicians or physician substitutes. Their authority derives from nursing education, nursing certification, and nursing licensure—applied within appropriate specialty boundaries.

This distinction has historical precedent. Peplau's psychiatric nursing theory demonstrated that specialty-focused nursing practice could maintain nursing identity while incorporating specialized knowledge from psychology and psychiatry. Her nurses practicing psychotherapy were not becoming psychologists; they were applying psychological knowledge through a nursing framework (Peplau, 1952; Peplau, 1997). Similarly, contemporary specialty-certified nurse practitioners apply specialty medical knowledge through a nursing framework, maintaining their professional identity while exercising specialized expertise.

7. CONSULTATION, COLLABORATION, AND RECOGNITION OF LIMITS

Autonomous practice includes the professional obligation to recognize the limits of one's expertise and to consult or refer when patient needs exceed one's scope. A family nurse practitioner working in a specialty clinic should:

- Practice within FNP scope for routine matters
- Consult with or refer to specialty-certified providers (physician specialists, specialty-certified NPs) for complex specialty-specific decisions
- Engage in ongoing education but not assume specialty scope without appropriate certification
- Maintain transparency with patients about their qualifications and scope

This is not a limitation of autonomy but an expression of professional responsibility. Autonomous practice means exercising independent judgment within one's scope—not practicing without boundaries.

8. EMERGING SPECIALTY NP ROLES

Some nurse practitioner specialties continue to emerge through formal education programs and certification pathways:

- Oncology nurse practitioners with specialized oncology certification
- Cardiology nurse practitioners with advanced cardiac training and certification
- Orthopedic nurse practitioners with musculoskeletal specialty preparation
- Emergency nurse practitioners with emergency certification
- Dermatology nurse practitioners with dermatology certification

These roles are legitimate expressions of Specialty Care (Domain 5) when supported by appropriate education, certification, and competency validation. As nursing education continues to evolve, additional specialty pathways may emerge—always grounded in nursing's distinct professional framework.

9. SUMMARY OF SCOPE PRINCIPLES

Within nursopathic medicine:

- Autonomous practice requires alignment between education, certification, and clinical scope
- Employment setting does not expand scope of practice
- Nurse practitioners practice **as nurse practitioners** in specialty areas, not as physician subspecialists
- Specialty practice follows nursing's population- and context-focused model, not medicine's organ-system model
- Professional responsibility includes recognizing limits and consulting appropriately
- Emerging specialty roles are legitimate when supported by formal education and certification

These principles protect patients, preserve professional integrity, and ensure that autonomous practice remains grounded in competence and accountability.

Table 12.1. Employment Setting vs. Scope of Practice: Critical Distinction.

Employment Setting	Scope Of Practice
Where you work	What you're certified to do
Changes with job	Determined by education + certification
Employer-determined	Certification board-determined
Variable	Stable unless recertified
Example: Cardiology clinic	Example: Family NP (FNP-C)
✘ Does NOT expand scope	✔ Defines autonomous authority

An FNP employed in cardiology practices AS AN FNP in that setting—not as a cardiology specialist. Scope follows certification, not employment.

10. POPULATION-FOCUSED EXPERTISE

Specialization in advanced nursing practice is grounded in population-focused education and training. Nurse practitioners develop deep familiarity with the physiologic, psychological, developmental, or procedural characteristics that distinguish their specialty populations.

This expertise informs assessment, diagnosis, and management by allowing nuanced interpretation of clinical findings within a defined context. Specialty-specific knowledge enhances precision without altering the underlying structure of autonomous practice.

11. ADVANCED ASSESSMENT AND DIAGNOSTIC REASONING

Within specialty practice, assessment extends beyond general evaluation to include advanced interpretation of findings that may be subtle, atypical, or highly context-dependent. Nurse practitioners apply refined diagnostic reasoning shaped by repeated exposure to specialty-specific presentations and trajectories.

This domain emphasizes that diagnostic authority within nursing is not diluted by specialization, but rather strengthened through focused experience and expertise.

12. INTEGRATION OF SPECIALTY KNOWLEDGE INTO AUTONOMOUS DECISIONS

Specialty Care requires the integration of focused knowledge into independent clinical decision-making. Nurse practitioners must translate specialty evidence, standards, and evolving practices into individualized care plans while maintaining accountability for outcomes.

Within the nursopathic framework, this integration reinforces autonomy by aligning specialized expertise with independent authority rather than deferring decision-making based on role hierarchy.

13. MAINTAINING COHERENCE ACROSS DIVERSE PRACTICE ROLES

As nurse practitioners practice across increasingly diverse settings and specialties, maintaining coherence in professional identity becomes essential. Specialty Care preserves coherence by anchoring specialization within a shared framework of reasoning, accountability, and evidence-based practice.

This domain affirms that specialization represents variation in focus, not variation in legitimacy or authority.

14. INTEGRATION WITH OTHER DOMAINS

Specialty Care integrates specialized knowledge across all other domains. Acute Care is enhanced by specialty-specific pattern recognition, Chronic Care by population-focused longitudinal management strategies, Preventative Care by specialty-appropriate risk assessment, and Interdisciplinary Care by expertise-based consultation and referral.

15. DURABILITY ACROSS SETTINGS AND SPECIALTIES

Specialty Care is durable across clinical environments because it is defined by function rather than title or task. Whether practiced in primary care, psychiatry, acute care, procedural settings, or subspecialty roles, specialization enhances autonomous practice without redefining its foundational structure.

16. ILLUSTRATIVE EXAMPLES ACROSS SPECIALTIES

- **Psychiatric-Mental Health NP:** Advanced psychiatric assessment, psychopharmacologic expertise, and specialized psychotherapeutic interventions for mental health populations.
- **Adult-Gerontology Acute Care NP:** Management of complex multisystem illness in high-acuity settings, including critical care and progressive care environments.

- **Women's Health NP:** Specialty care focused on reproductive and gynecologic health across the lifespan, including contraceptive management and menopausal care.
- **Neonatal NP:** Advanced physiologic management of critically ill neonates, including respiratory support and hemodynamic stabilization.
- **Orthopedic NP:** Specialty assessment and management of musculoskeletal conditions, including pre- and post-operative care.
- **Oncology NP:** Cancer-specific diagnostic and therapeutic expertise, including chemotherapy management and symptom palliation.

CHAPTER SUMMARY

Specialty Care within nursopathic medicine represents the focused expression of autonomous nursing authority. By situating specialization within a unified framework of clinical reasoning and accountability, this domain affirms that diversity in practice strengthens, rather than fragments, the professional identity of nurse practitioners.

CHAPTER 12
PRACTICE QUESTIONS

MULTIPLE CHOICE QUESTIONS

1. **Specialty Care in nursopathic medicine is defined by:**
   A. Employment setting
   B. Population- or condition-focused expertise informing advanced practice within defined domains
   C. Years of experience
   D. Hospital privileges

2. **Scope alignment requires that autonomous specialty practice be exercised within:**
   A. Any specialty where employed
   B. The specialty for which formally educated and nationally certified
   C. Any area after 5 years experience
   D. Whatever the employer requests

3. **An FNP employed in a cardiology clinic:**
   A. Automatically becomes a cardiology specialist
   B. Practices as an FNP within FNP scope in that setting
   C. Gains cardiologist scope
   D. Is no longer practicing nursing

4. **The distinction between employment setting and practice scope is critical because:**
   A. It affects salary
   B. Scope is determined by certification, not employment
   C. It determines parking privileges
   D. Settings don't matter

5. **Legitimate specialty practice requires:**
   A. Only employment in that specialty
   B. Graduate education, national certification, and documented competency in that specialty
   C. Physician approval
   D. Five years of experience

6. **Nursing's approach to specialty practice is:**
   A. Organ-system focused like medicine
   B. Population- and context-focused
   C. Identical to physician subspecialties
   D. Unorganized

7. **When a specialty-certified NP (e.g., oncology NP) practices in their specialty, they are:**
   A. Becoming physicians
   B. Applying specialty medical knowledge through a nursing framework
   C. Abandoning nursing
   D. Practicing medicine illegally

8. **Consultation, collaboration, and recognition of limits are:**
   A. Signs of incompetence
   B. Professional obligations in autonomous practice
   C. Unnecessary with certification
   D. Only for new graduates

9. Population-focused expertise in Specialty Care includes:

A. Only demographic data

B. Deep familiarity with physiologic, psychological, developmental, or procedural characteristics of specialty populations

C. Marketing to specific groups

D. Geographic location

10. The professional obligation to consult or refer when patient needs exceed one's scope is:

A. A limitation of autonomy

B. An expression of professional responsibility

C. Admission of incompetence

D. Unnecessary for experienced NPs

CASE-BASED APPLICATION QUESTIONS

Case Scenario 1:

An FNP is offered a high-paying position in an orthopedic surgery practice managing complex pre- and post-operative patients. The role includes managing post-surgical complications and advanced musculoskeletal assessments—topics not covered in FNP preparation.

Questions:

- What questions must be addressed before accepting this position?
- Why doesn't employment in the orthopedic setting expand the NP's scope?
- What would constitute appropriate preparation for this role?

Case Scenario 2:

An experienced oncology NP with formal oncology certification states, "I practice medicine in my specialty area—I manage complex cancer treatments, adjust chemotherapy, handle complications. But I'm doing this AS A NURSE PRACTITIONER, not trying to be an oncologist. What's the difference?"

Questions:

- Using Chapter 12's framework, explain what makes her practice distinctly nursing despite managing complex oncology.
- How does nursing's population-focused approach differ from medicine's organ-system focus?
- Why is this distinction professionally important?

TRUE/FALSE SELF-ASSESSMENT

1. ______ Specialty Care is defined by employment setting.
2. ______ An FNP working in cardiology automatically gains cardiology specialist scope.
3. ______ Legitimate specialty practice requires formal education and certification in that specialty.
4. ______ Consultation and referral are signs of incompetence.
5. ______ Recognition of limits is an expression of professional responsibility, not a limitation of autonomy.

See Appendix B for complete answers and rationales.

PART IV

SYNTHESIS AND IMPLICATIONS

CHAPTER 13

ETHICAL FOUNDATIONS OF NURSOPATHIC MEDICINE

LEARNING OBJECTIVES

Upon completing this chapter, students will be able to:

Explain why ethics applies to practice design and institutional structures, not just individual decisions.

Articulate the principle that authority and responsibility must be aligned for ethical practice.

Describe accountability as a patient-safety obligation rather than punitive measure.

Analyze why role clarity is an ethical requirement, not just operational preference.

Distinguish between ethical collaboration (clear boundaries, mutual respect) and confused roles.

Evaluate how transparency and trust depend on legible, explainable systems.

Apply ethical principles to assess whether practice structures support or undermine patient-centered care.

CRITICAL THINKING QUESTIONS

Institutional Ethics: The chapter focuses on ethics at the level of practice design rather than bedside decisions. Provide an example of a system or institutional structure that creates ethical problems even when individual clinicians act in good faith.

Authority-Responsibility Alignment: You're held accountable for patient outcomes but required to get physician approval for routine clinical decisions you're educated and certified to make. Using this chapter's framework, explain why this is an ethical problem, not just an inconvenience.

Moral Distress: The chapter treats moral distress as "a diagnostic signal" of system failure. Describe a situation where you or an NP you know experienced moral distress. What misalignment between authority and responsibility caused it? How could the system be redesigned ethically?

Role Clarity vs. Flexibility: Some argue that rigid role boundaries limit collaboration and flexibility in dynamic healthcare environments. Others argue clarity prevents confusion and error. Construct both sides of this debate using the ethical framework from this chapter. Which is more convincing?

Evaluation: The chapter states it "evaluates structures, not people" and doesn't "assess professional worth" or "rank disciplines." Why are these distinctions important? How does focusing on structures rather than individuals change the ethical analysis?

Application: You're designing a new urgent care clinic staffed by NPs, PAs, and MDs. Using this chapter's ethical principles (authority-responsibility alignment, accountability, role clarity, transparency), how would you structure the practice?

Reflection: Have you encountered a situation where practice structure (policies, hierarchies, approval processes) created ethical problems separate from individual behavior? How might the principles in this chapter have helped address it?

1. INTRODUCTION

Healthcare ethics is often discussed at the bedside, focusing on individual decisions, consent, and professionalism. While these matters remain essential, many of the most significant ethical risks in modern healthcare arise not from individual behavior, but from practice structures and systems (Grace, 2018). Who holds authority, who bears respon-sibility, and how accountability is assigned are ethical questions before they are clinical ones.

Nursopathic medicine is built on the premise that practice architecture matters ethically. This chapter establishes the ethical foundations that guide the design of roles, responsibilities, and systems throughout this book. It focuses on institutions and professional structures, not individual moral character or clinical judgment.

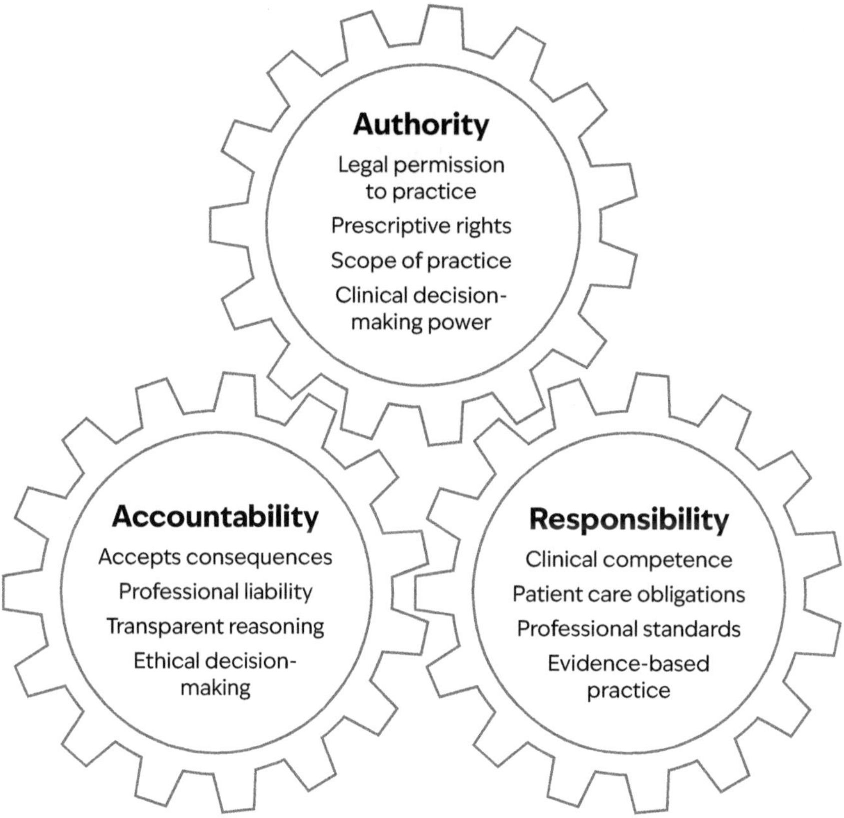
Authority
Legal permission to practice
Prescriptive rights
Scope of practice
Clinical decision-making power
Accountability
Accepts consequences
Professional liability
Transparent reasoning
Ethical decision-making
Responsibility
Clinical competence
Patient care obligations
Professional standards
Evidence-based practice

✓ **Aligned:** Authority + Responsibility + Accountability = Ethical Autonomous Practice

✗ **Misaligned:** Authority without Accountability = Potential for harm

✗ **Misaligned:** Accountability without Authority = Cannot act on clinical judgment

Figure 13.1. Ethical Foundation: Alignment of Authority, Responsibility, and Accountability

2. ETHICS AT THE LEVEL OF PRACTICE DESIGN

Clinical ethics traditionally addresses what a clinician ought to do in a particular situation. Institutional ethics asks a different question: Are the systems within which clinicians work ethically sound?

Practice models, scope definitions, and care pathways shape behavior long before any individual decision is made. When authority is unclear, accountability diffuses. When responsibility is misaligned with decision-making power, patient safety is compromised (Kohn et al., 2000; Institute of Medicine, 2011).

For this reason, nursopathic medicine treats ethics as a design requirement, not an afterthought.

3. AUTHORITY AND RESPONSIBILITY MUST BE ALIGNED

A core ethical principle of this framework is that authority and responsibility must travel together (Beauchamp & Childress, 2019; Grace, 2018).

- Authority without responsibility invites risk
- Responsibility without authority creates moral distress
- Clear alignment protects patients, clinicians, and systems

Ethically sound systems ensure that clinicians who make decisions are the same clinicians who are accountable for outcomes. This principle is foundational to patient safety, professional integrity, and public trust (Beauchamp & Childress, 2019).

Nursopathic medicine therefore rejects models in which decision-making authority is separated from clinical responsibility by formality alone.

4. ACCOUNTABILITY AS A PATIENT-SAFETY OBLIGATION

Accountability is not punitive. It is protective.

Patients deserve to know:

- Who is responsible for their care
- Who is making decisions
- How those decisions are governed

From an ethical standpoint, accountability is owed first to the patient, not to professional hierarchy or tradition. Systems that obscure accountability (through layered permissions, indirect authority, or unclear supervision) place unnecessary burden on patients and clinicians alike.

Ethically robust practice models make accountability visible, direct, and understandable.

5. ROLE CLARITY IS AN ETHICAL REQUIREMENT

Ambiguous roles are often defended as flexible or collaborative. In practice, they are a common source of error, delay, and conflict.

Role clarity:

- Reduces cognitive load
- Improves coordination
- Supports safe delegation
- Strengthens interdisciplinary trust

From an ethical perspective, role clarity respects both patients and professionals. It allows each clinician to practice within a defined scope, with appropriate authority and responsibility, without hidden dependencies.

Nursopathic medicine treats role clarity as a moral obligation, not merely an operational preference.

6. COLLABORATION WITHOUT CONFUSION

Ethical collaboration does not require blurred roles. It requires mutual respect within clear boundaries.

Interdisciplinary care is strongest when:

- Each discipline's expertise is recognized
- Decision-making authority is explicit
- Responsibility is not diluted by committee or hierarchy

This framework supports collaboration at clearly defined interfaces, where expertise is exchanged without transferring accountability away from the clinician responsible for care.

Collaboration enhances ethics when it clarifies responsibility, not when it conceals it.

7. TRANSPARENCY AND TRUST

Trust in healthcare depends on transparency. Patients, families, and institutions must be able to understand how decisions are made and who is responsible for them.

Ethically sound systems:

- Make decision pathways visible
- Avoid unnecessary complexity
- Do not rely on informal workarounds

Transparency is not about exposure; it is about legibility. Systems that can be explained clearly are more likely to be trusted, defended, and sustained.

8. ETHICS, REGULATION, AND PROFESSIONAL IDENTITY

This chapter distinguishes ethics from regulation:

- Ethics asks whether a system is fair, safe, and justifiable
- Regulation determines how authority is formally assigned

Ethics does not assume that existing regulations are optimal. It provides a framework for evaluating whether regulatory structures support or undermine patient-centered care, professional accountability, and system stability.

Importantly, this ethical framework:

- Does not assess professional worth
- Does not rank disciplines
- Does not argue clinical superiority
- It evaluates structures, not people.

9. INSTITUTIONAL ETHICS AND MORAL DISTRESS

When clinicians are held responsible without commensurate authority, moral distress follows. Persistent moral distress is not merely an individual burden; it is a sign of ethical system failure (Hamric, 2012)

Nursopathic medicine treats moral distress as a diagnostic signal:

- A mismatch between authority and responsibility
- A breakdown in role clarity
- A failure of institutional ethics

Ethically sound systems minimize moral distress by aligning expectations with actual control.

10. BOUNDARIES OF THIS ETHICAL FRAMEWORK

This chapter does not:

- Replace nursing or medical ethics codes
- Dictate individual clinical decisions
- Resolve all ethical disagreements

Its purpose is narrower and more structural:

- To define ethical guardrails for practice design
- To clarify how authority, responsibility, and accountability should relate
- To prepare the reader for later analysis of regulation and justice

Clinical Reflection: When Licensure and Practice Authority Diverge

I remember transitioning to a new position after having worked as an experienced nurse practitioner in urology—both inpatient and outpatient—for over a year. I accepted what I thought would be an advancement: a role working alongside another urologist.

Despite holding an autonomous license in Florida and having practiced independently in my previous position, my role in this practice was structured as clinical support rather than independent practice. My responsibilities centered on documentation, message management, and assisting with procedures—functions that utilized my clinical knowledge but not my autonomous diagnostic and therapeutic authority.

This experience illustrated the misalignment of authority, responsibility, and accountability described in this chapter. I held legal authority to practice independently under state law. I bore professional responsibility for patient outcomes when I did contribute to clinical decisions. Yet the employment structure granted me limited actual decision-making power, creating a disconnect between regulatory authority and practice reality.

Clinical disagreements revealed this structural challenge most clearly. For instance, my approach to managing hyperestrogenism in patients on testosterone replacement therapy—prescribing anastrozole based on evidence and my prior successful management—differed from the physician's preference to avoid intervention. It is worth noting that testosterone replacement therapy and its associated management—including monitoring for hyperestrogenism and prescribing aromatase inhibitors such as anastrozole—falls within FNP scope and is routinely addressed in primary care settings. PMHNPs encounter it as well, given testosterone's documented effects on mood, cognition, and psychiatric symptom presentation. My authority to manage this was not derived from working in a urology clinic; it was part of my FNP scope that I brought into that setting.

This wasn't necessarily a matter of one approach being wrong and another right. It was a situation where two clinicians with overlapping clinical authority held different evidence-based perspectives, yet the employment structure lacked a framework for understanding how my autonomous clinical judgment operated within that setting.

The physician likely understood my role through the traditional employment model he had experienced: nurse practitioners function as physician extenders, their clinical judgment operating under physician direction. This wasn't malicious—it was the default model in the absence of a clear alternative framework. Without a conceptual understanding of nurse practitioner practice as autonomous medicine practiced through a nursing lens, the structure reverted to familiar hierarchical patterns.

I eventually left for a primary care position where I could practice autonomously again, and I remained there until obtaining my psychiatric-mental health nurse practitioner certification and starting my own practice.

Before I left, however, I encountered a situation that underscored the importance of professional boundaries and accountability. The clinic director asked me to send six months' worth of prescriptions to patients so the physician would have fewer administrative tasks after my departure. I was pressured to comply despite my objections. I refused. Years earlier, in a different practice, I had done exactly that—pre-signed prescriptions for continuity after my departure—and was later subpoenaed by an attorney who claimed I was prescribing to his client long after I had left the practice. The legal and professional risk was clear. This time, I stood firm.

What these experiences taught me was that autonomous practice authority at the state regulatory level doesn't automatically translate to autonomous practice structure at the employment level—and more fundamentally, that professional accountability extends beyond employment relationships and organizational convenience. I remained legally and ethically responsible for prescriptions bearing my signature long after leaving that practice. The alignment of authority and accountability isn't just about structural coherence—it's about ethical integrity and patient safety.

This experience exemplifies the ethical dimensions of autonomous practice described in this chapter. The misalignment of authority, responsibility, and accountability created not just structural confusion but ethical dilemmas. The employment structure granted me responsibility for patient outcomes while limiting my authority to make independent clinical decisions—a situation that made ethical practice difficult if not impossible.

The prescription signing incident demonstrates that professional accountability extends beyond employment relationships. I remained legally and ethically responsible for prescriptions bearing my signature long after leaving that practice. When the clinic director pressured me to pre-sign six months of prescriptions for organizational convenience, refusing was not just a professional boundary—it was an ethical requirement. Exercising prescriptive authority requires ongoing clinical judgment, patient monitoring, and the ability to adjust or discontinue medications based on changing clinical circumstances. Pre-signing prescriptions without that ongoing accountability would have been ethically indefensible, regardless of organizational convenience.

This illustrates why the alignment of authority and accountability is fundamentally an ethical requirement, not just an operational preference. When employment structures grant responsibility without corresponding authority, or when pressure exists to exercise authority without maintaining accountability, ethical practice becomes impossible. The framework this chapter describes—that authority, responsibility, and accountability must be aligned—is not just about professional autonomy. It's about the ethical coherence required for responsible patient care.

Autonomous practice, properly understood, includes clear accountability. The prescription incident taught me that autonomous authority comes with sustained responsibility. I could not ethically sign prescriptions for patients I would no longer monitor, evaluate, or be available to. That lesson—that authority and accountability are inseparable—is central to understanding nursopathic medicine as an ethical framework, not just a practice model.

CHAPTER SUMMARY

Nursopathic medicine rests on a simple ethical premise: patients are safest when authority, responsibility, and accountability are aligned within transparent systems. Ethics in this framework is not aspirational rhetoric but practical discipline applied to how care is organized. By grounding practice design in clear ethical principles, the framework supports patient trust, professional integrity, and sustainable systems of care.

CHAPTER 13
PRACTICE QUESTIONS

MULTIPLE CHOICE QUESTIONS

1. **The ethical foundation of autonomous practice rests on:**
   A. Regulatory permission
   B. Alignment of authority, responsibility, and accountability
   C. Physician delegation
   D. Years of experience

2. **When authority is present but accountability is absent, the result is:**
   A. Autonomous practice
   B. Ethical misalignment and potential for unchecked harm
   C. Appropriate delegation
   D. Collaborative practice

3. **Beneficence in autonomous NP practice requires:**
   A. Following protocols without deviation
   B. Clinical competence and commitment to evidence-based standards
   C. Always deferring to physicians
   D. Avoiding difficult decisions

4. **Nonmaleficence ("first, do no harm") includes responsibility to:**
   A. Avoid treating complex patients
   B. Recognize limits and seek consultation when appropriate
   C. Never make mistakes
   D. Practice defensively

5. **Patient autonomy in shared decision-making means:**
   A. Patients make all decisions alone
   B. NPs provide evidence-based guidance respecting patient values and preferences
   C. NPs decide what's best
   D. Following family wishes over patient wishes

6. **Justice in nursopathic medicine addresses:**
   A. Legal compliance only
   B. Equitable access to competent autonomous care
   C. Billing practices
   D. Hierarchies between providers

7. **Professional integrity requires:**
   A. Never admitting uncertainty
   B. Honest acknowledgment of limits, appropriate consultation, and ethical decision-making
   C. Appearing confident at all times
   D. Practicing beyond scope to meet patient needs

8. **The relationship between authority and accountability is:**
   A. Optional based on setting
   B. Inseparable, authority without accountability is ethically unsustainable
   C. Determined by regulations
   D. Relevant only for physicians

9. **Ethical autonomous practice requires:**
   A. Complete independence from all others
   B. Competence, humility, and commitment to patient welfare over ego
   C. Advanced degrees only
   D. Working in independent practice settings

10. When NPs encounter situations beyond their scope or competence, ethical practice requires:

A. Proceeding anyway to meet patient expectations

B. Consultation, referral, or acknowledgment of limitations

C. Hiding uncertainty

D. Pretending competence

CASE-BASED APPLICATION QUESTIONS

Case Scenario 1:

A newly graduated FNP is offered full practice authority in a state with independent practice. She has strong didactic knowledge but limited clinical experience. The job offers excellent pay and no supervision requirement.

Questions:

- How does the alignment of authority-responsibility-accountability apply to this situation?
- What ethical obligations does she have despite having legal authority?
- How should she approach the transition to independent practice ethically?

Case Scenario 2:

An experienced NP encounters a patient with a rare presentation outside their usual scope. The patient has difficulty accessing specialists and asks the NP to manage the condition because "you're just as good as any doctor."

Questions:

- What ethical principles are in tension here?
- How does professional integrity guide the response?
- What would constitute an ethical approach to this situation?

TRUE/FALSE SELF-ASSESSMENT

1. ______ Authority without accountability is ethically appropriate if regulations allow it.
2. ______ Professional integrity requires honest acknowledgment of limits.
3. ______ Beneficence means always giving patients what they want.
4. ______ Justice in nursopathic medicine addresses equitable access to competent autonomous care.
5. ______ Ethical practice requires perfection and never making mistakes.

See Appendix B for complete answers and rationales.

CHAPTER 14

JUSTICE, REGULATION, AND THE DESIGN OF PRACTICE AUTHORITY

LEARNING OBJECTIVES

Upon completing this chapter, students will be able to:

Explain Rawlsian justice principles and their application to institutional structures (using the call-out box as reference).

Distinguish between evaluating regulatory structures versus evaluating individual clinicians or professions.

Compare independent and restrictive practice authority models using justice principles.

Analyze how regulatory design affects access, opportunity, and accountability in healthcare.

Apply the difference principle (inequalities justified only if they benefit the least advantaged) to practice authority.

Evaluate whether various regulatory approaches are publicly justifiable and transparent.

Synthesize understanding of how regulation constitutes part of healthcare's basic institutional structure.

CRITICAL THINKING QUESTIONS

Veil of Ignorance: Use Rawls thought experiment: If you didn't know whether you'd be a patient in a rural area, an NP, a physician, or a person with limited healthcare access, would you prefer independent or restrictive practice authority? Construct your reasoning.

Objections: The chapter anticipates several objections to its analysis (restrictive models enhance safety, historical precedent justifies hierarchies, autonomy is zero-sum, etc.). Choose one objection and develop it fully. Then respond using the chapter's framework. Which side is more convincing?

International Application: Apply Rawlsian analysis to one international regulatory model from Chapter 6/Appendix A. Is that structure more or less just than U.S. models? Use specific principles from this chapter.

Access and Justice: The chapter connects practice authority to access for underserved populations. Research your state or region: Are there areas where restrictive NP regulation limits access? How would you make a justice-based (not just utilitarian) argument for regulatory change?

Transparency: The chapter emphasizes that just institutions must be "publicly justifiable" and transparent. Find your state's NP practice act. Is it transparent and easily explainable to citizens? If not, what creates opacity?

Critical Evaluation: This chapter takes a normative stance that restrictive models are "ethically difficult to justify." Do you find the argument convincing? What's the strongest counterargument? How would you respond to it?

Synthesis: Design a regulatory framework for advanced practice from scratch using Rawlsian principles. What would it look like? How would it handle scope, supervision, collaboration, and accountability? Justify each decision using justice principles.

1. INTRODUCTION

Regulation is not merely an administrative mechanism; it is a structural determinant of access, opportunity, and accountability within healthcare systems. State practice acts and licensure frameworks shape who may provide care, under what conditions, and with what responsibilities. As such, regulation constitutes part of the basic institutional structure of healthcare and is therefore an appropriate subject for ethical evaluation.

This chapter examines regulatory approaches to advanced practice authority through the lens of institutional justice, drawing on Rawlsian principles (Rawls, 1971) to assess whether existing structures are fair, publicly justifiable, and sustainable. The analysis focuses on systems, not individuals, and avoids claims about professional virtue or clinical superiority. Its purpose is to evaluate whether different regulatory environments align authority with function in a manner consistent with justice, transparency, and public trust (Safriet, 2011).

FOR READERS UNFAMILIAR WITH JOHN RAWLS

Who was John Rawls?

John Rawls (1921-2002) was a political philosopher best known for *A Theory of Justice* (1971). His work is widely used in ethics, law, and health policy to think about what makes institutions fair.

What Rawls is NOT used for in this book:

- He is not a guide for individual clinical decisions
- He does not replace nursing ethics or clinical judgment
- He is not a bedside moral algorithm

How Rawls IS used here:

- As a way to think about fair role design
- To guide how authority and accountability should be structured
- To avoid privileging professions based on power or tradition

Key idea in simple terms:

If you were designing a healthcare system without knowing what role you would occupy in it, you would likely favor clarity, fairness, and accountability. This book uses that insight to shape professional frameworks. Not personal behavior.

RAWLS KEY TERMS: QUICK REFERENCE GUIDE

To help readers follow the analysis in this chapter, here are Rawls key concepts defined in plain language:

- **Veil of Ignorance:** A thought experiment where you design rules for society without knowing what position you'll occupy in it (rich/poor, powerful/powerless, urban/rural, patient/provider). This prevents self-interest from shaping the rules. Applied here: Would you accept practice authority rules if you didn't know whether you'd be a patient needing care, an NP, a physician, or someone in an underserved area?
- **Difference Principle:** Inequalities (differences in power, authority, resources) are only just if they benefit the least advantaged members of society. Applied here: Restricting NP practice authority creates inequality (physicians have more authority than NPs). Is this justified? Only if it somehow benefits patients who are worst off (underserved populations). If it reduces access for vulnerable populations, it fails this test.
- **Original Position:** The hypothetical situation where people choose principles of justice behind the veil of ignorance, before knowing their place in society. Used to determine what rules rational people would accept as fair. Applied here: What practice authority rules would rational people choose if they didn't know their own role in the healthcare system?
- **Basic Structure:** Rawls focuses on the fundamental institutions and systems that shape society (laws, government, major social institutions), not individual actions. Applied here: Regulatory frameworks are part of healthcare's basic structure, they determine who can practice and under what conditions, affecting everyone's opportunities and access.

- **Public Justification:** Just institutions must be explainable and defensible to citizens in terms they can reasonably accept, not just through power or tradition. Applied here: Can restrictive practice authority rules be publicly justified? Can we explain why they're fair in terms the public would accept, or do they rely on professional self-interest?
- **Reflective Equilibrium:** The process of adjusting our principles and judgments until they cohere, when our moral intuitions match our considered principles. Applied here: Testing whether our gut reactions about practice authority align with principles of justice we'd accept more generally.
- **Justice as Fairness:** Rawls overall theory name, the idea that justice means fairness in how society's basic structure is organized, ensuring equal liberties and fair opportunities for all.
- **Liberty Principle:** Everyone should have equal basic liberties (freedom, opportunity to participate). Applied here: Do qualified NPs have equal opportunity to practice their profession, or do regulatory structures unfairly constrain their liberty compared to other professionals with similar preparation?
- **Fair Equality of Opportunity:** Jobs and positions should be open to all based on talent and effort, not arbitrary barriers. Applied here: If NPs are educated, certified, and competent, should they face arbitrary practice restrictions that aren't based on patient safety evidence?
- **Least Advantaged:** People in society who are worst off, those with fewest opportunities, resources, or power. In healthcare, this often means people in rural areas, low-income communities, or underserved populations who face the greatest barriers to accessing care.

How to use these terms: As you read the chapter, when you encounter one of these concepts, refer back to this box. The analysis will make more sense once you understand what these terms mean and how they apply to practice authority.

Remember: Rawls isn't being used here to judge individual people or professions, but to evaluate whether regulatory systems are designed fairly.

This chapter evaluates regulatory structures, not individual clinicians, professions, or patient care decisions. It does not argue for or against any professional group's competence, nor does it assess clinical outcomes.

The ethical framework used here applies principles of justice to institutions and policies, consistent with established approaches in healthcare ethics. Readers should not interpret this analysis as commentary on bedside decision-making or professional motivation.

Disagreement with the conclusions is reasonable. The purpose of the chapter is to make the ethical reasoning behind regulatory design explicit and open to scrutiny.

2. REGULATION AS AN ETHICAL STRUCTURE

Healthcare regulation distributes power. It determines who can act, who must defer, and who bears responsibility for outcomes. These distributions are not value-neutral; they reflect assumptions about competence, trust, risk, and legitimacy.

Rawls theory of justice is particularly relevant because it treats justice as a property of institutions, not of individual moral character. From this perspective, the ethical question is not whether clinicians act in good faith, but whether the rules governing practice can be reasonably accepted as fair by those subject to them.

In healthcare, where access delays, workforce shortages, and inequities disproportionately affect vulnerable populations, regulatory design has direct moral consequences.

3. RAWLSIAN JUSTICE IN PLAIN TERMS

Rawls proposes that fair institutions are those that rational persons would accept if they did not know what position they themselves would occupy within the system. This is illustrated by the veil of ignorance, a thought experiment intended to prevent self-interest from shaping institutional rules (Rawls, 1971, 1993).

Applied to healthcare regulation, the question becomes:

> *Would a rational person accept these rules governing practice authority if they did not know whether they would be a patient, a clinician, or a member of an underserved community?*

This chapter applies Rawls narrowly and deliberately:

- Only to institutional design
- Not to individual clinical decisions
- Not to professional worth or identity

This limited use is consistent with contemporary applications of Rawls in health policy ethics.

4. PRACTICE AUTHORITY AS INSTITUTIONAL DESIGN

Practice authority determines how care is delivered, not just who delivers it. When authority is aligned with licensure, training, and accountability, systems tend toward clarity and stability. When authority is contingent on external permission unrelated to function, systems introduce friction, dependency, and opacity.

From a Rawlsian standpoint, the ethical evaluation of practice authority turns on several questions:

- Is opportunity distributed fairly among qualified professionals?
- Does the structure benefit the least advantaged?
- Are the rules transparent and publicly justifiable?
- Is the system stable over time?

These questions apply regardless of profession.

5. INDEPENDENT AND RESTRICTIVE PRACTICE ENVIRONMENTS

Variation among U.S. states provides a natural comparison of regulatory models. As of 2024, over thirty states and the District of Columbia have enacted full practice authority legislation permitting nurse practitioners to practice independently (AANP, 2024).

- **Independent practice environments** grant nurse practitioners authority aligned with licensure and scope, holding them directly accountable for care.
- **Restrictive environments** condition practice on mandated supervisory or collaborative arrangements, regardless of context or competence.

This chapter does not presume intent or motivation. Many restrictive frameworks arose from historical compromise rather than ethical deliberation. Nevertheless, Rawlsian analysis evaluates outcomes of structure, not origins.

Table 14.1. Comparison of Regulatory Models for Nurse Practitioner Practice.

Feature	Full Practice Authority	Reduced Practice	Restricted Practice
Physician Oversight	None required	Career-long collaborative agreement	Supervision/delegation required
Prescriptive Authority	Independent	Independent with collaborative agreement	Delegated or limited
Diagnostic Authority	Independent	Independent with collaboration requirement	Supervised
Practice Location	Any appropriate setting	Any setting with collaborating physician	Physician-supervised settings
Patient Outcomes	Equivalent to physician care	Equivalent to physician care	No evidence of superior outcomes

Feature	Full Practice Authority	Reduced Practice	Restricted Practice
Healthcare Access	Improved access, especially underserved areas	Moderate access barriers	Significant access barriers
Number of States (2026)	30+ states + DC	~15 states	~5 states
Justice Analysis	Supports equitable access	Creates unnecessary barriers	Worsens healthcare inequities

Note. Data adapted from American Association of Nurse Practitioners (2024).

6. JUSTICE, ACCESS, AND THE LEAST ADVANTAGED

Rawls difference principle holds that inequalities are justified only if they benefit the least advantaged members of society. In healthcare, the least advantaged are often those facing geographic, economic, or systemic barriers to care.

Regulatory structures that limit the effective supply of qualified clinicians. By tying practice authority to availability of supervisors rather than patient need, risk exacerbating access gaps. Conversely, structures that align authority with function are more likely to expand access without diluting accountability. This is not speculative. A systematic review of advanced practice nurse outcomes spanning nearly two decades found that nurse practitioners deliver care comparable to or exceeding that of physicians across multiple quality measures, with no evidence that restrictive oversight models produce superior patient safety (Newhouse et al., 2011). The Institute of Medicine's landmark report on the future of nursing documented geographic and population-specific access failures directly linked to state-level practice restrictions, particularly in rural and underserved communities (Institute of Medicine, 2011). Primary care workforce analysis has shown that nurse practitioner autonomy represents one of the most viable pathways for addressing shortages in areas where physician supply is insufficient

(Naylor & Kurtzman, 2010). If the least advantaged populations, those in rural areas, low-income communities, and underserved regions, do not benefit from restrictive practice authority, and the evidence suggests they are harmed by it, the difference principle is not satisfied.

This is not an argument about professional superiority; it is an argument about institutional efficiency and fairness.

7. TRANSPARENCY, TRUST, AND PUBLIC JUSTIFICATION

Rawls emphasizes that just institutions must be publicly justifiable, their rules should be explainable in terms that citizens can reasonably accept.

Transparency is central to this legitimacy. In healthcare, transparency underpins trust among patients, clinicians, and the public. High-functioning systems make clear who is responsible for decisions, how evidence is used, and how collaboration occurs.

Contemporary work on clinical evidence emphasizes that transparency and shared responsibility are foundational to societal trust and effective decision-making (Kohn et al., 2000). Regulatory models that obscure accountability or diffuse responsibility through contractual dependencies risk undermining this trust.

8. INTERDISCIPLINARY CARE AND REGULATORY ALIGNMENT

Modern healthcare increasingly depends on interdisciplinary and transdisciplinary collaboration to address complex problems. Research across diverse fields demonstrates that integration of expertise, rather than hierarchical control, supports innovation, quality, and equity (WHO, 2010; IPEC, 2016; Reeves et al., 2017).

Interdisciplinary collaboration functions best when authority and responsibility are clear. Regulatory structures that fragment authority can complicate collaboration by introducing ambiguity about decision-making and accountability. This insight aligns with broader concerns in health research and clinical implementation that conceptual vagueness and misaligned roles impede effective collaboration.

As discussed in Chapter 11 (Interdisciplinary Care), collaboration is most effective at a well-defined interdisciplinary interface. This chapter asks whether regulation enables that clarity or undermines it.

9. SHARED DECISION-MAKING AND PATIENT INTERESTS

Patient-centered care relies on shared decision-making, which requires time, trust, and clear clinician accountability. Effective shared decision-making acknowledges power asymmetries and emphasizes transparency, deliberation, and responsibility.

Regulatory environments that complicate clinician accountability or constrain continuity of care can inadvertently burden patients, particularly those navigating complex or chronic conditions. From a Rawlsian perspective, institutional arrangements should protect patients from avoidable complexity created by professional regulation rather than clinical necessity.

10. STABILITY AND SUSTAINABILITY

Rawls argues that just institutions must be stable, they must generate their own support over time without constant enforcement. Regulatory systems that rely on workaround arrangements, contractual supervision, or informal delegation may function, but they do so at the cost of clarity and sustainability.

As healthcare systems face demographic shifts, workforce shortages, and increasing complexity, regulatory adaptability becomes an ethical concern. Structures that align authority with competence are more likely to remain stable and responsive over time.

11. ANTICIPATED OBJECTIONS AND SCHOLARLY DIALOGUE

This chapter's application of Rawlsian justice to regulatory structures will invite critique, as all normative ethical arguments do. Some may argue that:

- **Restrictive models enhance patient safety through oversight** (though outcome data increasingly challenge this assumption, and oversight can occur through other accountability mechanisms)
- **Historical precedent justifies current hierarchies** (though history alone is insufficient ethical justification, particularly when circumstances have changed substantially)
- **Professional autonomy for one group diminishes another** (though this assumes a zero-sum rather than collaborative model of interdisciplinary practice)
- **This analysis privileges individual liberty over collective goods** (though Rawlsian justice explicitly considers benefits to the least advantaged, not merely individual freedom)

These objections deserve serious engagement. This chapter offers one ethical framework (Rawlsian institutional justice) as a lens for evaluating regulatory design. Other ethical approaches (utilitarian calculations of outcomes, virtue ethics focusing on professional character, communitarian emphasis on collective goods, or care ethics emphasizing relationships) might yield different conclusions or emphasize different values.

The purpose here is not to foreclose debate but to elevate it, to move regulatory discussions beyond workforce arguments and professional turf battles toward principled ethical reasoning about fair institutional design. Whether one accepts these specific conclusions, the method of subjecting regulatory structures to ethical scrutiny strengthens healthcare governance and advances professional discourse.

Nursing scholarship benefits when theoretical frameworks engage with difficult normative questions. This chapter invites response, refinement, and continued dialogue about how healthcare authority should be justly structured in service of patients and communities.

Reflective Note: Why Rawlsian Justice in a Nursing Theory Framework?

This chapter has examined nurse practitioner regulation through the lens of Rawlsian justice, applying principles like the veil of ignorance, fair equality of opportunity, and the difference principle to scope of practice debates. The choice to use this particular philosophical framework was not arbitrary or merely academic—it emerged from a long intellectual journey that began well before my nursing career.

Isaac Newton wrote in 1675 to Robert Hooke, "If I have seen further it is by standing on the shoulders of Giants." (Newton, 1675) This work stands on the shoulders of philosophical traditions that have profoundly shaped our understanding of justice and human rights. John Locke's conviction that governments exist by the consent of the governed to protect natural rights to life, liberty, and property laid groundwork that John Rawls would later refine through his theory of justice as fairness (Locke, 1689/1980). Both thinkers have shaped foundational frameworks for equitable governance and fair treatment—principles as essential to healthcare regulation as to political philosophy.

Clinical Reflection: Justice as a Lens—How Rawls Shaped My Understanding of Nursing Practice

I first encountered John Rawls during undergraduate studies in an introductory philosophy course. There I was exposed to various philosophical traditions (utilitarianism, Kantian ethics, social contract theory), but two thinkers proved particularly influential: John Locke and John Rawls. Rawls A Theory of Justice fundamentally shaped how I understood fairness, particularly as it applies at the institutional and structural level rather than merely at the level of individual action.

I was especially drawn to Rawls principle of justice as fairness and his thought experiment of the "veil of ignorance." The concept is elegant: rational people designing a just society would do so from behind a veil of ignorance, not knowing what position they themselves would occupy in that society. Without knowing whether they would be rich or poor, powerful or marginalized, majority or minority, they would design institutions that are fair from every position because any position might be theirs.

The green vine spiraling through the Interdisciplinary Care column carries additional meaning: it is a homage to Rawls veil of ignorance, that thought experiment in which we design systems not knowing our own position within them. The vine's measured balance—neither constricting nor fumbling—mirrors the veil's demand that we create structures fair to all, regardless of where we might find ourselves within them.

What struck me as I progressed through nursing education and into nurse practitioner practice was how persistently institutional arrangements in healthcare seemed to favor existing power structures. Healthcare professionals across all disciplines naturally tend toward positions that align with their training, experience, and professional identity. This is human nature, not a unique failing of any particular profession. When physicians express concerns about nurse practitioner scope expansion, those concerns often reflect multiple legitimate considerations: patient safety based on their understanding of appropriate training and supervision, preservation of care quality standards they were trained to uphold, and understandable concern about how evolving professional boundaries might affect their own practice patterns and professional roles.

I observed this dynamic clearly in scope of practice debates. The challenge from a justice perspective is not that physicians hold these positions—it would be surprising if they didn't, given human tendencies toward maintaining familiar structures and protecting established roles. The challenge is that institutional arrangements, once established, tend to perpetuate themselves even when the original justifications may no longer align with current evidence or changing healthcare needs.

Research on nurse practitioner practice outcomes has accumulated substantial evidence over decades, generally showing that autonomous NP practice in primary care and other settings produces patient outcomes comparable to physician care in similar contexts (Newhouse et al., 2011). This evidence base suggests that at least some scope restrictions may no longer be supported by patient safety data, even if they once reflected reasonable caution about a newer professional role.

I realized that Rawls veil of ignorance provided a powerful analytical tool not for assigning blame, but for examining structural fairness. If we designed healthcare regulatory structures without knowing which profession we would occupy—physician, nurse practitioner, physician assistant, pharmacist, patient—would we choose the current system? Would we design institutions that grant one profession supervisory authority over another based not on individual competency assessment but on historical precedent? Would we create barriers that limit access to care in underserved areas to preserve traditional professional hierarchies?

The answer, I believe, depends on whether current arrangements serve demonstrable patient benefit or persist primarily through institutional inertia. From behind the veil of ignorance, rational actors would likely design healthcare institutions based on principles of fair equality of opportunity and arrangements that benefit patients, particularly those with least access to care. They would ask: Do these regulations improve patient outcomes? Do they enhance access to care for underserved populations? Do they distribute opportunity fairly among qualified professionals?

This realization was reinforced by a conversation with a DO colleague who had previously worked as a physician assistant. She described the frustration of being highly trained and clinically competent yet systematically positioned in a subordinate role—not because of demonstrated deficiency in clinical judgment, but because of regulatory and institutional arrangements that assumed hierarchical relationships regardless of individual competence. Her experience illustrated how professional boundaries based on credential rather than demonstrated competency can feel arbitrary to those affected, even when those boundaries were established with legitimate concerns about quality and safety.

Rawls framework provides conceptual tools to argue that some regulatory restrictions may not withstand scrutiny under principles of justice as fairness. This doesn't require assuming bad faith or attributing mercenary motives to anyone. It simply provides a method for asking whether the rules we've inherited still serve their intended purposes, or whether they persist more from path dependency than from current evidence of benefit.

This framework allows us to separate legitimate patient safety concerns—which deserve serious consideration and evidence-based evaluation—from institutional inertia or arrangements that may serve professional interests more than patient welfare. It doesn't assume bad faith. It provides analytical tools for distinguishing between regulations that demonstrably protect patients and regulations that primarily protect existing professional structures.

This is why Rawlsian justice appears in this chapter and throughout this book. It is not a weapon against physicians or any other profession. It is a rigorous analytical framework for evaluating whether healthcare institutions are structured in ways that serve justice and patient welfare, or whether they preserve arrangements that made sense historically but may no longer align with current evidence about how healthcare can best be delivered.

> *This chapter's application of Rawlsian principles to nurse practitioner regulation demonstrates how philosophical frameworks can illuminate structural issues that remain obscured when debates focus only on individual competencies or professional loyalties. The veil of ignorance, as applied here, doesn't question anyone's motivations—it questions whether institutional arrangements that may have made sense historically still serve their stated purposes today.*
>
> *By examining regulatory structures through principles of justice as fairness, this chapter invites all healthcare professionals—physicians, nurses, administrators, policymakers—to*

consider whether current arrangements would be chosen if designed without knowing which role one would occupy. This isn't about winning a professional turf war. It's about asking whether the rules governing advanced practice serve the principles of fair opportunity and patient benefit that would be chosen from behind the veil of ignorance.

Philosophy was my first love, long before nursing. This reflective note is, I confess, a love letter to that discipline—an attempt to bring rigorous ethical reasoning into a field that desperately needs clear normative frameworks. If Rawls theory of justice as fairness can illuminate and transcend this discussion of nurse practitioner autonomy, then perhaps this framework honors not only his contribution but also the patients and practitioners whose lives depend on just, defensible systems of care.

The analytical tools Rawls provides—distinguishing just institutions from those that preserve existing advantages, evaluating whether inequalities benefit the least advantaged, ensuring arrangements are publicly justifiable—offer a way to evaluate scope of practice regulations without assuming bad faith from anyone. They simply ask: Are these arrangements just? This chapter demonstrates that for many restrictions on autonomous nurse practitioner practice, the answer may be no.

CHAPTER SUMMARY

This chapter has examined practice authority as a matter of institutional justice, not professional advocacy. Using Rawlsian principles as a normative yardstick, it suggests that regulatory environments aligning authority with licensure, function, and accountability are more easily justified in terms of fairness, transparency, and sustainability. Restrictive regulatory structures are not portrayed as malicious or irrational but shown to be ethically difficult to justify under widely accepted principles of institutional justice, particularly when they limit access, obscure accountability, or disadvantage those already underserved. This analysis situates regulation firmly within the ethical architecture of nursopathic medicine.

CHAPTER 14
PRACTICE QUESTIONS

MULTIPLE CHOICE QUESTIONS

1. **Rawlsian justice, as applied to NP practice, emphasizes:**
   A. Market forces
   B. Fair equality of opportunity and benefit to the least advantaged
   C. Maximizing revenue
   D. Professional hierarchies

2. **The "veil of ignorance" thought experiment asks:**
   A. Whether NPs remember their training
   B. What regulatory system one would choose without knowing their position within it
   C. Whether patients understand provider roles
   D. How to hide credentials

3. **The "difference principle" suggests regulatory restrictions are justified only if they:**
   A. Increase physician income
   B. Benefit the least advantaged or improve overall access to care
   C. Reduce NP practice
   D. Maintain traditional hierarchies

4. **When regulatory restrictions fail to improve patient access or outcomes, they represent:**
   A. Appropriate caution
   B. Justice concern, barriers serving professional protection rather than public welfare
   C. Evidence-based policy
   D. Standard practice

5. **Justice analysis asks whether restrictive practice regulations:**
   A. Protect physician employment
   B. Actually serve their stated purpose (patient safety) or primarily benefit incumbent professionals
   C. Increase complexity
   D. Preserve tradition

6. **Fair equality of opportunity in healthcare access means:**
   A. Everyone gets the same treatment
   B. Qualified professionals can practice to full scope without arbitrary barriers
   C. Market competition
   D. Urban-focused care

7. **When evidence shows autonomous NP practice is safe but restrictions remain, this suggests:**
   A. Evidence doesn't matter
   B. Possible regulatory capture, protectionism rather than public welfare
   C. Appropriate caution
   D. Scientific uncertainty

8. **The justice framework for evaluating scope restrictions asks:**
   A. Do they protect existing practitioners' market share?
   B. Do they improve access for underserved populations?
   C. Do they increase bureaucracy?
   D. Do they follow tradition?

9. **Nursopathic medicine's justice argument emphasizes:**
   A. NP superiority
   B. That autonomous practice can address healthcare access inequities
   C. Eliminating physicians
   D. Deregulation for economic benefit

10. **From a justice perspective, requiring collaboration agreements without evidence they improve outcomes:**
   A. Is prudent policy
   B. Creates barriers that may worsen access for vulnerable populations
   C. Protects patients
   D. Is standard practice

CASE-BASED APPLICATION QUESTIONS

Case Scenario 1:

A rural county has high maternal mortality and no obstetricians. Women's health NPs could provide prenatal care, but state law requires physician collaboration. The nearest collaborating physician is 120 miles away and unwilling to supervise remotely. Pregnant women must travel 3+ hours for care or go without.

Questions:

- Apply the Rawlsian "difference principle", do collaboration requirements benefit the least advantaged here?

- What does the "veil of ignorance" reveal about this regulatory structure?
- How does this illustrate justice concerns with restrictive practice regulations?

Case Scenario 2:

In State A (independent practice), rural and underserved populations have good NP access. In State B (restrictive), these populations have worse access despite similar NP workforce. Physician organizations in State B argue restrictions "ensure quality," but outcomes data shows no safety difference.

Questions:

- What justice issue does this comparison reveal?
- How does Rawlsian analysis apply when restrictions don't improve outcomes but worsen access?
- What questions should policymakers ask from a justice perspective?

TRUE/FALSE SELF-ASSESSMENT

1. ______ The "veil of ignorance" asks what system we'd choose without knowing our position in it.
2. ______ Restrictive regulations are automatically justified if they claim to protect safety.
3. ______ The difference principle says restrictions are just only if they benefit the least advantaged.
4. ______ Justice analysis examines whether regulations serve public welfare or incumbent professional interests.
5. ______ Access to care is unrelated to justice concerns in NP regulation.

See Appendix B for complete answers and rationales.

CHAPTER 15

CONCLUSION—A COHERENT FRAMEWORK FOR AUTONOMOUS NURSING PRACTICE

LEARNING OBJECTIVES

Upon completing this chapter, students will be able to:

Synthesize the complete nursopathic medicine framework, including all five domains and their integration, into a coherent explanation of autonomous nurse practitioner practice.

Explain why autonomous practice is an ethical and structural necessity that emerges logically from the responsibilities nurse practitioners already carry, rather than an aspirational goal awaiting expanded authority.

Analyze the relationship between responsibility, authority, and ethical coherence, and explain why fragmented authority undermines both patient safety and professional integrity.

Evaluate the claim that autonomy is the condition under which evidence-based practice can be applied responsibly and consistently, and articulate how constrained authority interferes with evidence-based care.

Describe the implications of the nursopathic medicine framework for nursing education, clinical practice, and professional regulation.

Apply the framework to emerging challenges in advanced practice nursing, including technology integration, international expansion, and scholarly development.

Reflect on how the nursopathic medicine framework addresses the conceptual gap identified in Chapter 1 and articulate what the profession gains from a nursing-centered explanation of autonomous practice.

CRITICAL THINKING QUESTIONS

Synthesis: The chapter argues that autonomous practice is a "structural and ethical necessity" rather than an aspiration. Trace this argument through the preceding chapters: How does each chapter build toward this conclusion? What would healthcare delivery look like if this necessity went unacknowledged?

Responsibility Without Authority: Describe a situation where a nurse practitioner is held responsible for patient outcomes but lacks commensurate authority to make clinical decisions. Using this chapter's framework, explain why this arrangement is ethically untenable and what patient and professional harms may result.

Evaluation: The chapter claims autonomous practice "emerges logically from the responsibilities already assumed within advanced nursing practice" rather than requiring expanded authority. Do you find this framing persuasive? Why might this distinction matter for professional and policy discussions?

Full Circle: Return to Chapter 1's problem statement. How does nursopathic medicine address the conceptual gap between regulatory recognition and theoretical explanation? What does the framework provide that was previously missing, and what work remains?

Application: You are designing a new NP program or revising an existing curriculum. How would you use the five-domain model to structure clinical rotations, learning objectives, and competency assessments differently than traditional setting-based approaches? Be specific about what would change and why.

Reflection: How has your understanding of what "autonomy" means changed through reading this book? What did you believe it meant before? What do you understand it to mean now, and what practical difference does that shift make?

Debate: Critics argue that autonomous NP practice is justified only in areas with physician shortages, not in urban centers where physicians are available. Using the necessity and ethical coherence arguments from this chapter, explain why the "shortage-only" framing is both theoretically insufficient and practically harmful.

1. PURPOSE AND SCOPE

This concluding chapter serves a dual purpose: it synthesizes the complete nursopathic medicine framework and it makes the case that autonomous nurse practitioner practice is not an aspirational goal awaiting permission, but a structural and ethical necessity that emerges directly from the responsibilities advanced practice nurses already carry.

Rather than defining practice through tasks, settings, or comparisons, the model articulates the functional domains through which advanced nursing authority is exercised. In doing so, it offers a coherent explanation of how nurse practitioners reason, act, and remain accountable across diverse clinical contexts. That coherence is not only theoretically satisfying—it is ethically required. When responsibility is present, authority must follow.

The purpose of this framework is not to redefine scope or advocate for structural change, but to clarify the internal logic of advanced nursing practice as it exists. By naming and organizing the functions of practice, nursopathic medicine provides a shared professional language capable of supporting education, regulation, and interdisciplinary collaboration.

2. AUTONOMOUS PRACTICE AS ETHICAL AND STRUCTURAL NECESSITY

Autonomous nurse practitioner practice is not optional. It is not a workforce accommodation for underserved areas, a temporary measure in the face of physician shortages, or a professional preference to be weighed against organizational convenience. It is a necessity—structural because the healthcare system cannot meet its obligations without it, and ethical because the responsibilities already borne by nurse practitioners demand commensurate authority.

This chapter makes that argument explicitly. Each preceding chapter has built toward it: the conceptual gap identified in Chapter 1, the historical precedent established in Chapter 2, the framework defined in Chapters 3 through 6, the five domains elaborated in Chapters 7 through 12, and the ethical and justice analyses of Chapters 13 and 14. Together, they do not merely describe what nurse practitioners do—they demonstrate why autonomous practice is the only arrangement that is coherent, safe, and just.

2.1 Responsibility, Authority, and Ethical Coherence

Nurse practitioners routinely assume responsibility for clinical assessment, diagnosis, management, and outcomes across diverse settings (Institute of Medicine, 2011; Fairman et al., 2011). The ethical principle that follows is equally clear: responsibility must be paired with commensurate authority (Beauchamp & Childress, 2019). When authority is withheld or mediated despite sustained accountability, clinicians are placed in ethically untenable positions—held responsible for outcomes over which they have only partial control. This misalignment is not merely inefficient; it is a structural ethical failure.

Autonomous practice resolves this misalignment by ensuring that those responsible for outcomes possess the authority to make and revise clinical decisions. Within nursopathic medicine, autonomy is not independence from collaboration, but independence of judgment within collaborative systems.

2.2 Accountability as the Foundation of Autonomy

Autonomy within nursopathic medicine is inseparable from accountability. Nurse practitioners are accountable to patients, regulatory bodies, and professional standards for the outcomes of their clinical decisions. This accountability presupposes the ability to exercise judgment without unnecessary external constraint.

Fragmented authority obscures accountability by diffusing responsibility across roles. When decision-making authority requires external approval, the chain of accountability becomes difficult to trace. Autonomous practice restores clarity by locating decision-making authority with the clinician who bears responsibility for outcomes—a transparency that is not only organizationally useful but a patient safety imperative.

2.3 Continuity of Care and Patient Safety

The five domains established in this text—Acute Care, Chronic Care, Preventative Care, Interdisciplinary Care, and Specialty Care—describe how nurse practitioner practice spans time, acuity, and specialization. Fragmentation of authority across these domains disrupts continuity of care and undermines patient safety.

Autonomous practice enables coherent clinical reasoning across time and settings. It allows nurse practitioners to integrate acute responses, preventive strategies, and specialty knowledge into unified care plans without reliance on external authorization that may delay or dilute clinical decisions.

2.4 Evidence-Based Practice and Professional Judgment

Autonomy does not imply deviation from evidence-based standards—on the contrary, it requires rigorous adherence to scientific evidence, clinical guidelines, and professional norms (Sackett et al., 1996; Melnyk & Fineout-Overholt, 2019). Within nursopathic medicine, autonomy is the condition under which evidence-based practice can be applied responsibly and consistently, rather than selectively or indirectly. When a clinician must seek approval before implementing an evidence-based intervention, the gap between evidence and action introduces risk. Autonomous practice closes that gap by placing the decision where the evidence and the accountability converge—with the clinician responsible for the patient.

2.5 The Structural Necessity Argument

Beyond individual clinical encounters, autonomous NP practice is a structural necessity for the healthcare system itself. The United States faces chronic shortages of primary care and psychiatric providers, disproportionately affecting rural, low-income, and underserved populations (Naylor & Kurtzman, 2010; National Governors Association, 2012). An aging population with increasing chronic disease burden requires longitudinal, relationship-based care that nurse practitioners are trained and equipped to provide.

Decades of research demonstrate that NP care produces outcomes comparable to or exceeding those of physician care across a wide range of conditions and settings (Newhouse et al., 2011). Restrictive practice regulations have not been shown to improve patient outcomes, but have consistently been shown to reduce access, particularly for vulnerable populations (Safriet, 2011). Healthcare cost pressures require the full and efficient utilization of all qualified professionals—constraining NP practice to less than full scope wastes trained capacity the system cannot afford to waste.

The argument is not that nurse practitioners should replace physicians. It is that a healthcare system that does not fully utilize its autonomous NP workforce fails patients measurably—in access gaps, in delayed diagnoses, and in underserved populations who receive no care at all.

2.6 Autonomy Within Interdisciplinary Systems

Autonomous practice functions within, not outside of, interdisciplinary healthcare systems. Collaboration enhances care by integrating diverse expertise, but collaboration does not require subordination of professional judgment (IPEC, 2016). Effective interdisciplinary teams are built on clarity about each member's autonomous authority, not on hierarchical permission structures. By clarifying authority and accountability, autonomous practice strengthens interdisciplinary relationships and reduces role ambiguity, enabling nurse practitioners to contribute fully as accountable clinicians rather than conditional participants.

3. REAFFIRMING THE PURPOSE OF NURSOPATHIC MEDICINE

This book has advanced nursopathic medicine as a unifying framework for understanding autonomous nurse practitioner practice. The five domains—Acute Care, Chronic Care, Preventative Care, Interdisciplinary Care, and Specialty Care—are not discrete silos. They represent interdependent dimensions of a single professional role. Together, they describe how nurse practitioners assume responsibility for patient outcomes across time, acuity, and specialization.

- **Acute Care** addresses moments of instability and uncertainty, requiring rapid assessment, probabilistic reasoning, and decisive action under time constraints.
- **Chronic Care** sustains responsibility beyond episodic encounters, demanding longitudinal reasoning, pattern recognition across time, and deliberate management of evolving conditions.
- **Preventative Care** anticipates and mitigates foreseeable harm, embedding risk reduction as a core clinical obligation rather than a discrete service line.
- **Interdisciplinary Care** integrates diverse professional expertise while preserving autonomous authority, recognizing that collaboration and autonomy are complementary, not contradictory.
- **Specialty Care** refines expertise without fragmenting professional identity, applying population-specific knowledge within the same ethical and epistemological framework that grounds all five domains.

Their integration reflects the continuity and accountability that define autonomous practice. All five domains rest upon the foundation of Evidence-Based Practice, ensuring that autonomy is exercised within established scientific and professional standards. The architectural model introduced in Chapter 7—five equal columns of white marble supporting a unified pediment—conveys this integration visually: no single domain stands above the others, and none can be removed without compromising the whole.

4. AUTONOMY AS ALIGNMENT, NOT ISOLATION

Throughout this text, autonomy has been framed as the alignment of authority, responsibility, and accountability—not as independence from collaboration. Nurse practitioners practice autonomously within interdisciplinary systems, exercising independent judgment while engaging team-based care to enhance patient outcomes.

By locating autonomy within ethical and structural coherence, nursopathic medicine reframes longstanding debates. Autonomy is not a privilege to be granted or withheld based on professional politics or historical convention. It is a condition required for responsible clinical practice when sustained accountability is present. The practitioner who bears responsibility for a patient's diagnosis, treatment, and outcomes must possess the authority to make and revise those decisions. This is not a claim for expanded power—it is a description of what ethical practice requires.

5. IMPLICATIONS FOR EDUCATION, PRACTICE, AND REGULATION

A shared framework for nurse practitioner practice carries implications beyond theory.

For education, nursopathic medicine supports curricular coherence by organizing competencies around functional domains rather than fragmented tasks. Programs can structure learning objectives, clinical experiences, and assessments around the five domains, ensuring graduates are prepared not only to perform clinical tasks but to assume full professional responsibility within scope. The five domains can serve as organizing principles for curriculum development, clinical competency assessment, and continuing education, with clear progression from foundational knowledge to autonomous practice.

For practice, the framework clarifies role expectations and strengthens interdisciplinary integration. Nurse practitioners can articulate their practice more clearly to patients, colleagues, and institutions. The framework reduces ambiguity about what nurse practitioners do and how their authority functions, providing language for conversations that previously had no shared vocabulary.

For regulation, it provides a neutral language that emphasizes accountability, patient safety, and evidence-based decision-making without redefining scope. Regulators can use this framework to evaluate competence, guide policy development, and support public understanding without requiring uniform statutory language. As more states move toward independent practice models, the framework provides a theoretical foundation explaining why such models align with nursing education, ethics, and accountability structures.

6. LOOKING FORWARD: FUTURE DIRECTIONS

Autonomous practice by nurse practitioners will continue to evolve in response to changes in healthcare delivery, population needs, and clinical complexity. The purpose of nursopathic medicine is not to predict specific regulatory or professional outcomes, but to provide a stable conceptual framework capable of accommodating future developments without undermining professional identity or accountability.

6.1 Expansion Across Settings and Specialties

As practice environments diversify, the need for a unifying explanation of autonomous practice becomes more pronounced. Nursopathic medicine offers such an explanation by identifying common structures of reasoning, responsibility, and collaboration that transcend specialty boundaries. This coherence allows autonomous practice to adapt while remaining conceptually grounded.

6.2 Evolution of Educational Standards

As clinical expectations increase, educational programs will need to emphasize advanced reasoning, diagnostic accuracy, and longitudinal management. Nursopathic medicine provides a framework for aligning curricular goals with practice realities, ensuring that graduates are prepared not only to perform clinical tasks but to assume full professional responsibility within scope.

6.3 Regulatory Consistency and Clarity

Future regulatory discussions are likely to focus on consistency, transparency, and public understanding of professional roles. By offering a nursing-centered language for autonomous practice, nursopathic medicine may support clearer communication between regulators, policymakers, and the public—reducing misinterpretation and fostering trust without requiring changes to existing regulatory structures.

6.4 Enhanced Interdisciplinary Integration

Interdisciplinary collaboration will continue to be a defining feature of healthcare. Nursopathic medicine situates collaboration within autonomy, recognizing that independent authority and teamwork are not mutually exclusive. Future work should explore how nurse practitioners can most effectively engage with emerging healthcare roles and how interdisciplinary education can prepare all professions for collaborative practice within clearly defined scopes.

6.5 Scholarly Development and Empirical Validation

Future scholarship will be essential to refining and evaluating the nursopathic model. Questions for future investigation include: How does education organized around the five domains affect clinical competence and professional identity? What outcomes are associated with practice in independent versus restrictive regulatory environments when controlling for other variables? How does the nursopathic framework translate across international contexts with different regulatory structures? By inviting scholarly engagement, nursopathic medicine positions itself as an evolving theory rather than a fixed doctrine, capable of growth as practice continues to change.

6.6 Technology and Innovation

The integration of technology in healthcare—including telehealth, artificial intelligence, and clinical decision support—will shape future practice. Nursopathic medicine's emphasis on clinical reasoning and accountability provides a framework for evaluating how technology enhances or challenges autonomous practice. Technology that supports diagnostic reasoning, longitudinal monitoring, and risk stratification will strengthen the domains; technology that displaces clinical judgment without equivalent accountability structures must be approached critically.

6.7 Global Perspectives and International Expansion

As advanced practice nursing continues to grow globally, nursopathic medicine offers a framework adaptable to diverse international contexts. While developed primarily from U.S. experience, the five-domain model applies wherever nurse practitioners or advanced nurse practitioners practice autonomously. The functional organization transcends jurisdiction-specific titles and regulatory language. Comparative studies examining how the five domains function across countries could strengthen theoretical understanding and inform regulatory development globally (Kleinpell et al., 2014; Delamaire & Lafortune, 2010).

Clinical Reflection: When the Vine Grows—Collaborative Relationships Built on Mutual Respect

Not all of my experiences with physician colleagues have involved conflict or structural barriers. I've had the privilege of working with excellent physicians who actively promoted nurse practitioner independence and understood autonomous practice as an asset rather than a threat. Two relationships stand out as examples of what interdisciplinary collaboration can look like when built on mutual professional respect.

The first was a physician colleague I met through the Direct Primary Care community. She was running her own small DPC practice while also expanding into professional coaching. We collaborated frequently—sometimes on clinical topics, more often on the business and operational challenges of independent practice. She genuinely admired what she described as my intelligence and marketing skills as a medical business owner, and she consistently encouraged me to use those abilities to help people. Our relationship wasn't hierarchical. We consulted as professional peers, each bringing different expertise and perspectives. When she had clinical questions, particularly about mental health, she asked for my input. When I had business or operational questions, she shared her experience generously.

What struck me most about this relationship was how natural it felt. There was no underlying tension about professional boundaries or scope of practice. She understood that my nurse practitioner practice was autonomous—that I practiced medicine through a nursing framework with independent clinical authority. That understanding didn't threaten her. It allowed us to collaborate productively because we both recognized the other's legitimate expertise and authority.

The second relationship was with my medical director while working in primary care for a multinational practice. She demonstrated what effective medical directorship looks like when it's understood as administrative coordination rather than clinical supervision. She listened to my perspectives on evidence-based practice changes—like the evolving guidelines on chlamydia treatment I had observed in my own patient outcomes. When clinical concerns arose, she treated my clinical reasoning as professional judgment deserving consideration, not subordinate opinion requiring approval.

Most significantly, when I obtained my autonomous license as a nurse practitioner and informed her I would no longer be signing a collaborative agreement, she was supportive and understanding. She recognized that my licensure granted me independent practice authority, and she respected that regulatory reality rather than treating it as an organizational inconvenience. Our working relationship didn't deteriorate—it simply shifted from a formal supervisory structure to professional collegiality.

These experiences taught me something important: when there is mutual respect and recognition of each profession's legitimate autonomous authority, collaboration enhances rather than constrains practice. Both of these physician colleagues understood intuitively what this framework articulates—that nurse practitioner practice is autonomous medicine practiced through a nursing lens, that it operates within a distinct professional framework while maintaining full diagnostic and therapeutic authority, and that this difference complements rather than replicates physician practice. They practiced the calibrated vine—neither too tight nor too loose—and everyone benefited.

These positive experiences don't erase the challenges described in earlier chapters. But they demonstrate that those challenges aren't inevitable. They emerge from structural and conceptual gaps—the absence of clear frameworks for understanding how autonomous nurse practitioner practice operates. When those frameworks exist, even informally through mutual understanding and professional respect, collaboration works. The vine supports growth.

CHAPTER SUMMARY

This chapter has accomplished two things simultaneously: it has made the case that autonomous nurse practitioner practice is an ethical and structural necessity, and it has synthesized the nursopathic medicine framework as the coherent explanation that practice has long required.

Autonomous practice is a necessity because responsibility already exists. Nurse practitioners already bear accountability for diagnoses, treatment decisions, and patient outcomes. Ethical coherence demands that authority match this responsibility. The healthcare system's access gaps, workforce realities, and documented outcomes data confirm what ethics requires: full utilization of the NP workforce, practicing to full scope, is not optional.

The nursopathic medicine framework organizes that practice into five functional domains—Acute Care, Chronic Care, Preventative Care, Interdisciplinary Care, and Specialty Care—supported by evidence-based practice and grounded in nursing's epistemology, ethics, and professional identity. These domains describe what nurse practitioners already do. The framework makes that practice legible, defensible, and teachable.

The conceptual gap that opened this book—the absence of a nursing-centered explanation for autonomous practice—has been addressed. Nursopathic medicine provides that explanation. The work now moves forward: refining the theory through scholarship, applying it in education, and using it to support clarity, accountability, and excellence in advanced nursing practice.

CLOSING STATEMENT

The collaborative relationships described in the preceding reflection exemplify what this framework enables when conceptual clarity supports practice. Autonomous nurse practitioner practice is best understood not through comparison or contention, but through the alignment of function, judgment, and accountability. Nursopathic medicine provides that alignment, offering a coherent and enduring framework for advanced nursing practice.

The five domains—Acute Care, Chronic Care, Preventative Care, Interdisciplinary Care, and Specialty Care—describe how nurse practitioners practice medicine through advanced nursing. These domains, supported by evidence-based practice, explain what nurse practitioners do, how they reason, and why their authority is not merely permitted but necessary for patient safety and system function.

By articulating nursopathic medicine, nursing gains a professional language for autonomous practice that is internally coherent, ethically sound, and adaptable to future evolution. This framework does not seek to displace other professions or claim superiority, but rather to clarify how nurse practitioners contribute to healthcare as accountable, autonomous clinicians practicing within nursing's traditions and values.

Nursing can and should explain its own most advanced practice through internally coherent, nursing-centered frameworks. This book offers that explanation. What happens next depends on whether the nursing profession, healthcare institutions, regulatory bodies, and our physician colleagues choose to recognize what already works and build systems that support it. Based on the relationships and experiences described throughout these pages, there is every reason to be hopeful that many will.

CHAPTER 15
PRACTICE QUESTIONS

MULTIPLE CHOICE QUESTIONS

1 **This chapter argues that autonomous NP practice is:**

A. Negotiable based on geographic setting

B. A structural and ethical necessity, not merely an aspirational goal

C. A luxury appropriate only for underserved areas

D. Controversial and unsupported by evidence

2 **The ethical case for autonomous practice rests primarily on:**

A. NP professional preferences

B. The principle that responsibility must be paired with commensurate authority

C. Economic competition with physicians

D. Regulatory convenience

3 **Fragmented authority across the five domains primarily undermines:**

A. Billing efficiency

B. Continuity of care and patient safety

C. Physician oversight mechanisms

D. Institutional hierarchy

4 **Autonomy within nursopathic medicine is defined as:**

A. Complete independence from all other professionals

B. Alignment of authority, responsibility, and accountability within collaborative systems

C. Freedom from regulatory oversight

D. The right to practice without consultation

5 **The structural necessity argument is supported by:**

A. Only anecdotal clinical reports

B. Workforce data, access inequities, cost pressures, and decades of safety and effectiveness research

C. Theoretical arguments alone

D. A single landmark study

6 **Autonomous practice and collaboration within nursopathic medicine:**

A. Are mutually exclusive

B. Coexist—autonomy of judgment operates within, not outside of, interdisciplinary systems

C. Require physician approval to function

D. Apply only in primary care settings

7 **The book's primary theoretical contribution is:**

A. Advocating for expanded NP scope of practice legislation

B. Explaining how NPs practice medicine through an advanced nursing framework

C. Proving NPs are clinically superior to physicians

D. Creating new licensure categories

8 **The five domains of nursopathic medicine represent:**

A. Sequential stages of career development

B. Functional dimensions of autonomous practice that operate together in every clinical encounter

C. Distinct service lines for different practice settings

D. Hierarchical levels of clinical authority

9 **The argument that autonomy is a "condition" for evidence-based practice means:**

A. Autonomous NPs create their own guidelines independent of evidence

B. When authority requires external approval before implementation, evidence-based interventions may be delayed or diluted

C. Evidence-based practice is only possible with physician oversight

D. Autonomous NPs ignore established clinical guidelines

10 **The book's ultimate message is that:**

A. NPs should transition to becoming physicians

B. Nursing can and should explain its own advanced practice through internally coherent, nursing-centered frameworks

C. Current autonomous practice is structurally unsustainable

D. Interdisciplinary collaboration should be eliminated

CASE-BASED APPLICATION QUESTIONS

Case Scenario 1:

A hospital system is struggling to staff ICUs and emergency departments. They have qualified ACNPs but regulations require physician supervision around the clock. Physicians are unavailable for overnight shifts. Administrators are considering reducing hours or closing units, leaving patients without access to care.

Questions:

- How does this scenario illustrate both the structural and ethical necessity arguments from this chapter?
- What are the access and safety implications of restrictive regulations in this case?
- How does the nursopathic framework explain why autonomous ACNP practice is the ethically coherent solution?
- What does this case reveal about the relationship between regulatory design and patient outcomes?

Case Scenario 2:

An experienced NP says: "I've been practicing for 15 years without needing a 'framework.' I just take care of patients. Why does this theoretical work matter?"

Questions:

- How would you explain the practical value of having an explicit theoretical framework beyond individual clinical competence?
- What can a shared professional framework accomplish that experience alone cannot?
- How does the nursopathic medicine model strengthen the profession beyond any single NP's practice?
- How does the framework address the imposter syndrome described in Chapter 1, and why does that matter professionally and clinically?

TRUE/FALSE SELF-ASSESSMENT

1. ______ The chapter argues that autonomous NP practice is optional and negotiable based on workforce conditions.
2. ______ Necessity is grounded in ethical coherence (authority must match responsibility) as well as system demands and research evidence.
3. ______ Autonomous practice is only structurally necessary in rural areas without physician coverage.
4. ______ Fragmentation of authority across the five domains can disrupt continuity of care and undermine patient safety.
5. ______ Restrictive practice regulations have been demonstrated to improve patient outcomes.

See Appendix B for complete answers and rationales.

APPENDICES

APPENDIX A

International Advanced Practice Nursing - Comparative Overview

Country	Title(s) Used	Education Requirements
United States	Nurse Practitioner (NP); subdivided by specialty (FNP, AGACNP, PMHNP, etc.)	Master's or Doctoral degree (MSN/DNP); national certification required
Canada	Nurse Practitioner (NP); may specify primary care or specialty	Master's degree (some provinces accepting post-RN certificate programs during transition); provincial/territorial registration
United Kingdom	Advanced Nurse Practitioner (ANP); Advanced Clinical Practitioner (ACP)	Master's-level education; no single national regulatory framework (profession-led)
Australia	Nurse Practitioner (NP)	Master's degree with advanced practice focus; national registration with endorsement
New Zealand	Nurse Practitioner (NP)	Master's degree in nursing; meets Nursing Council competencies; annual practicing certificate

This appendix provides a comparative overview of advanced practice nursing roles in selected countries. Information reflects general frameworks as of 2025; specific regulations may vary by region within countries and continue to evolve.

	Scope of Practice Summary	Autonomy Level	Year Established
	Full diagnostic, prescriptive, and management authority; scope varies by state	Varies by state: Full, Reduced, or Restricted practice authority	1960s
	Diagnostic, ordering tests, prescribing medications, performing procedures; scope and autonomy vary by province/territory	Varies by province: some grant full autonomy, others require collaborative agreements	1960s-1970s (expanded 1990s-2000s)
	Assessment, diagnosis, and treatment within clinical governance frameworks; prescribing with additional qualification	Collaborative practice within agreed protocols; varies by NHS trust and specialty	1990s-2000s (ongoing development)
	Autonomous practice including diagnosis, ordering investigations, prescribing medications, referring patients	Full practice authority within scope; Medicare rebates available	2000 (national framework established)
	Autonomous practice including assessment, diagnosis, prescribing, ordering tests, admitting/discharging patients	Full practice authority; can work independently	2001

Country	Title(s) Used	Education Requirements
Ireland	Advanced Nurse Practitioner (ANP)	Master's degree in advanced nursing practice; registration with NMBI (Nursing and Midwifery Board of Ireland)
Netherlands	Nurse Specialist (Verpleegkundig Specialist)	Master's-level education (2 years post-RN)
Sweden	Specialist Nurse (Specialistsjuksköterska); Advanced Practice Nurse (emerging)	Specialist nursing education (60-120 credits at master's level)
Norway	Advanced Practice Nurse (Avansert klinisk sykepleier - emerging role)	Master's degree in nursing; specialty certification
Finland	Clinical Nurse Specialist; Advanced Practice Nurse (emerging)	Master's degree; specialist certification
South Africa	Clinical Nurse Practitioner	Post-basic qualification (1-year program); registration with SANC within primary care scope

Scope of Practice Summary	Autonomy Level	Year Established
Autonomous clinical practice including assessment, diagnosis, and treatment, prescribing (with additional qualification)	Increasing autonomy; prescriptive authority established 2007; scope expanding	2001 (formally regulated)
Independent assessment, diagnosis, treatment, and prescribing within specialty areas; can admit/ discharge patients	High autonomy within defined specialty area; integrated into healthcare teams	1997 (formally recognized)
Advanced clinical practice in specialty areas; prescribing rights limited and varying by region	Variable; increasing movement toward greater autonomy	Specialty roles long-established; ANP concept emerging 2010s
Developing role with expanded assessment and limited prescribing in some areas	Evolving; varies by region and specialty	2010s (formal development ongoing)
Advanced clinical practice within specialty; prescribing rights limited	Variable; expanding in some healthcare districts	Specialist roles established; ANP framework emerging
Primary healthcare assessment, diagnosis, treatment, and prescribing within primary care scope	Autonomous within primary care scope; historically important for access in underserved areas	1970s-1980s

Notes:

- **Education:** Global trend toward master's-level preparation; some countries transitioning from certificate/diploma programs to graduate degrees
- **Terminology:** Titles vary but generally indicate autonomous advanced clinical practice with diagnostic and prescriptive authority
- **Regulation:** Some countries have national frameworks (Australia, New Zealand, Netherlands); others have regional variation (Canada, USA) or profession-led standards (UK)
- **Prescribing:** Most jurisdictions require additional qualification or registration for prescriptive authority beyond basic advanced practice license
- **Scope Variability:** Even within countries granting "full autonomy," practice may be limited by specialty, setting, or institutional policies
- **Evolution:** Many countries continue refining advanced practice frameworks; roles and regulations are dynamic

Applicability of Nursopathic Medicine Framework:

The five domains of nursopathic medicine (Acute Care, Chronic Care, Preventative Care, Interdisciplinary Care, and Specialty Care) apply across these international contexts regardless of specific titles or regulatory frameworks. Advanced practice nurses in all listed countries engage in:

- **Acute Care:** Managing urgent and time-sensitive clinical presentations
- **Chronic Care:** Longitudinal management of ongoing conditions
- **Preventative Care:** Health promotion, screening, and risk reduction
- **Interdisciplinary Care:** Collaboration with physicians and other healthcare professionals
- **Specialty Care:** Population- or setting-focused advanced practice

The universal applicability demonstrates that nursopathic medicine addresses fundamental aspects of advanced practice nursing that transcend national boundaries and regulatory structures.

Sources for Further Information:

- International Council of Nurses (ICN) - Guidelines on Advanced Practice Nursing
- World Health Organization - Resources on task-shifting and advanced practice roles
- Country-specific nursing regulatory bodies and professional organizations
- Academic literature on international advanced practice nursing development

Note: Readers should consult current regulatory authorities in specific jurisdictions for the most up-to-date information, as advanced practice nursing frameworks continue to evolve globally.

APPENDIX B

Practice Questions Answer Key

CHAPTER 1: THE PROBLEM OF AUTONOMOUS PRACTICE

Multiple Choice Answers

1. **B – The absence of theoretical explanation for how NPs practice medicine through nursing**

   Rationale: The conceptual gap is specifically defined as existing between regulatory recognition (NPs have legal authority) and theoretical explanation (lack of nursing-centered framework explaining HOW that authority functions). Option A addresses scope debates, Option C is unrelated to theory, and Option D concerns individual development rather than profession-wide conceptual needs.

2. **C – Alignment of authority, responsibility, and accountability**

   Rationale: The chapter defines autonomous practice as alignment of these three elements, ensuring the person making decisions is accountable for outcomes. Option A misunderstands autonomy as isolation. Option B confuses autonomy with absence of regulation. Option D contradicts the concept of inherent professional authority.

3. **B – Frame autonomy as contingent rather than inherent to advanced nursing practice**

   Rationale: The chapter explicitly states historical justifications are accurate but "have left autonomy interpreted as contingent rather than inherent," making them insufficient for explaining contemporary autonomous practice as a stable mode of advanced nursing. They're not inaccurate (A), and don't ignore safety (C) or focus too narrowly (D).

4. **B – The overlapping diagnostic and therapeutic authority exercised by NPs and physicians**

   Rationale: "Shared clinical space" is precisely defined as where NPs and physicians exercise overlapping diagnostic and therapeutic authority, creating conceptual tensions about professional boundaries. Not about physical space (A), meetings (C), or legal agreements (D).

5. **C – Provide a nursing-centered theoretical framework explaining autonomous practice**

   Rationale: The preface explicitly states this purpose, not advocacy for change (A), proving equivalence (B), or replacing theory (D). The book aims to explain existing practice, not expand or compare it.

6. **C – NPs experiencing doubt about professional legitimacy despite bearing full responsibility**

   Rationale: "Internalized uncertainty" refers to NPs experiencing doubt about professional legitimacy despite bearing full responsibility for clinical decisions and outcomes. A result of conceptual ambiguity. Not about exam anxiety (A), clinical skills (B), or specialty choice (D).

7. **B – How autonomous authority is understood**

   Rationale: The chapter explicitly states: "The central problem of autonomous practice, then, is not whether nurse practitioners are capable of independent clinical authority, but how that authority is understood." Focus is on theoretical understanding (B), not capability (A), regulation (C), or economics (D).

8. **B – Nurse practitioner practice at the APRN level**

   Rationale: Explicitly stated throughout: "Nursopathic medicine applies specifically to nurse practitioner practice at the advanced practice registered nurse level. It does not describe registered nursing practice." Not all nursing levels (A), only psychiatric (C), or educators (D).

9. **B – The practice domain of diagnosing and treating disease**

   Rationale: The chapter carefully defines medicine as "the systematic body of knowledge and clinical practice concerned with the diagnosis of disease and pathophysiological processes". A practice domain, not exclusive physician practice (A), only allopathic (C), or only hospitals (D).

10. **A – Assumption that autonomy already exists and needs explanation**

    Rationale: Focusing on "how" rather than "whether" assumes autonomous authority exists in practice and regulation, and needs theoretical explanation. Not avoidance (B), agreement with restrictions (C), or advocacy (D).

Case-Based Application - Suggested Answers

Case Scenario 1:

Question 1: Maria has full legal authority, appropriate education, and clinical competence, yet lacks theoretical language to explain HOW her practice functions within nursing. She can describe

WHAT she does (diagnose, prescribe, treat) but not WHY these activities constitute distinctly nursing-based autonomous practice. This perfectly illustrates the gap between regulatory recognition (she has it) and theoretical explanation (she lacks it).

Question 2: Maria may experience: (a) uncertainty about professional identity despite possessing full legal authority, (b) difficulty articulating her role in interdisciplinary relationships, (c) vulnerability to mischaracterization as a "physician substitute," and (d) internalized doubt about legitimacy despite bearing complete responsibility.

Question 3: Using nursopathic medicine, Maria could explain: "I practice medicine THROUGH a nursing framework. I'm educated in nursing, licensed as an advanced practice nurse, and accountable to nursing standards. My clinical reasoning integrates biomedical science with nursing's patient-centered, integrated approach. I exercise the same diagnostic and therapeutic authority, but through nursing's professional lens."

Case Scenario 2:

Question 1: Outcome data demonstrates WHAT NPs do and that care is safe/effective, but doesn't explain HOW NP practice fits conceptually within nursing or WHY NPs can practice medicine through nursing. Legislators' confusion is conceptual/theoretical, not empirical.

Question 2: The questions reveal the conceptual gap, lack of theoretical framework explaining the relationship between nursing professional identity and medical practice activities.

Question 3: Nursopathic medicine provides language: "NPs practice medicine through nursing, same diagnostic/therapeutic activities but through distinct professional framework, education, ethics, and accountability structures. This isn't physician substitution; it's nursing's highest level of autonomous practice."

True/False Answers

1. **FALSE** - The gap exists due to lack of theoretical explanation, not lack of clinical competence.
2. **FALSE** - Autonomy means alignment of authority, responsibility, and accountability, not isolation. Collaboration occurs within autonomous practice.
3. **TRUE** - Historical narratives are accurate but insufficient because they frame autonomy as contingent rather than inherent.
4. **FALSE** - Explicitly stated: applies only to NP practice at APRN level, not RN practice.
5. **TRUE** - Medicine is defined as the practice domain of diagnosing/treating disease, not exclusive to any profession.

CHAPTER 2: THE HISTORICAL DEVELOPMENT OF THE NURSE PRACTITIONER ROLE

Multiple Choice Answers

1. **B – Demonstrating that nurses could practice psychotherapy independently within a nursing framework, extending nursing rather than abandoning it**

   Rationale: Peplau's foundational contribution was demonstrating that psychiatric nurses could practice psychotherapy independently within a nursing framework — extending nursing rather than abandoning it. She did not create the first NP program (that came in the 1960s), nor did she establish prescriptive authority or make equivalence arguments.

2. **B – Nursing can integrate activities from other disciplines while maintaining professional identity**

   Rationale: Peplau established that nursing can integrate activities traditionally associated with other professions while maintaining its professional identity. This is the precedent that nursopathic medicine builds on directly: practicing medicine through nursing rather than becoming another profession.

3. **C – Master's-level education including supervised clinical practice**

   Rationale: Peplau insisted that advanced psychiatric nursing required master's-level education including supervised clinical practice in psychotherapy. She recognized that autonomous therapeutic practice required specialized graduate preparation — a principle that became foundational to all APRN education.

4. **B – Nurses practicing psychotherapy were extending nursing, not becoming psychologists**

   Rationale: "Role expansion without role abandonment" means that nurses practicing psychotherapy were extending the scope of nursing rather than abandoning nursing to become psychologists. This principle is directly applied in nursopathic medicine to NPs practicing medicine: expansion through nursing, not departure from it.

5. **B – Reinforces the perception that autonomy is contingent rather than inherent**

   Rationale: The chapter argues that grounding NP legitimacy in access, collaboration, or equivalence arguments inadvertently frames autonomy as contingent — something granted under certain conditions — rather than inherent to the NP's scope, education, and licensure. This leaves the profession theoretically vulnerable.

6. **C – History explains how the role developed, not how it currently functions as an autonomous clinical profession**

   Rationale: Historical narratives explain the circumstances that gave rise to the NP role but cannot explain how it currently functions as an autonomous clinical profession. History answers "how did this role come to exist?" — not "how does this practice operate as nursing?"

7. **B – Expanded to include diagnostic reasoning, pharmacology, and disease management alongside nursing theory**

   Rationale: As the NP role evolved, educational standards expanded to include diagnostic reasoning, pharmacology, and disease management alongside nursing theory. This reflects the increasing clinical authority NPs assumed over time, moving from delegated functions toward independent practice.

8. **B – The amplification of terms like "scope creep" and "dangerous" in media and social platforms that drown out substantive professional discourse**

   Rationale: The "echoes" refer to the amplification of adversarial terms — scope creep, dangerous, unqualified — across social media and news platforms in ways that drown out substantive professional discourse. The chapter argues the profession needs a theoretical voice capable of piercing that noise, not merely louder versions of the same pragmatic arguments.

9. **B - 1952**

   Rationale: Interpersonal Relations in Nursing was published in 1952. This is a factual anchor for the chapter — Peplau's foundational work predates the NP role by more than a decade, establishing the theoretical precedent before the practice role itself emerged.

10. **B – Nursopathic medicine addresses universal needs within nursing's evolution, not U.S.-specific circumstances**

    Rationale: The global emergence of advanced practice nursing roles — in the UK, Canada, Australia, New Zealand, and elsewhere — facing similar conceptual challenges suggests that the gap nursopathic medicine addresses is not a U.S.-specific phenomenon but a universal challenge in nursing's theoretical development.

Case-Based Application - Suggested Answers

Case Scenario 1:

Question 1: Peplau argued that psychiatric nurses practicing psychotherapy were not abandoning nursing for psychology. They were extending nursing through application of psychological knowledge within a nursing relational framework. She provided the theoretical structure that explained how the practice was distinctly nursing — grounded in nursing's interpersonal and therapeutic orientation — rather than a derivative of another profession.

Question 2: Peplau faced the claim that practicing psychotherapy meant practicing psychology — that the activity defined the profession. Sarah faces the same logic: that diagnosing and prescribing means practicing medicine in the physician sense. In both cases, the challenge confuses what is being done with who is doing it and through what professional framework. The activity does not determine the professional identity; the framework does.

Question 3: Sarah can explain that she is extending nursing — practicing psychiatric-mental health care through nursing's relational, patient-centered, and holistic orientation — not becoming a psychologist or physician. Her training, licensure, accountability, and epistemological grounding are all nursing. The diagnostic and therapeutic authority she exercises is nursing authority, grounded in advanced nursing education and national certification, not borrowed from another profession.

Case Scenario 2:

Question 1: History explains that NPs have safely provided care for 60+ years and that the role emerged from workforce needs. It does not explain what makes that practice nursing rather than medicine — which is the conceptual question the committee is actually asking. Outcome data and historical longevity cannot answer a question about professional identity and theoretical coherence.

Question 2: They are asking: what is the professional and theoretical basis for the clinical authority NPs exercise? History explains origin and precedent; it does not provide a framework explaining how diagnosing and treating illness is coherently nursing practice. That requires a theoretical model — which is precisely what nursopathic medicine provides.

Question 3: The scope of practice debate in public and legislative arenas is shaped by the loudest, most repeated claims — scope creep, safety concerns, professional hierarchy. A profession that can only respond with historical precedent and outcome studies is responding on the other side's terms. The echoes fill the room.

What the committee is implicitly asking for — and not receiving — is an internally coherent account of what NP practice is. That is the voice this book attempts to provide.

True/False Answers

1. **TRUE** - Peplau is widely recognized as the "mother of psychiatric nursing" for her foundational theoretical work on interpersonal relations in nursing and her advocacy for autonomous therapeutic practice by nurses.
2. **FALSE** - The NP role emerged from practical healthcare needs broadly, including primary care access in underserved settings — but framing it primarily as a response to physician shortages is an oversimplification. The chapter emphasizes that origin stories, however accurate, have limited explanatory power for what NP practice has become.
3. **TRUE** - Peplau insisted that advanced psychiatric nursing required master's-level education including supervised psychotherapy practice. This principle — that autonomous therapeutic authority requires graduate preparation — became foundational to all APRN education.
4. **TRUE** - This is the chapter's central argument about the limits of historical narrative: history explains the developmental trajectory of the NP role but cannot explain how that role currently functions as an autonomous clinical profession with its own theoretical basis.
5. **FALSE** - Peplau's framework was foundational but not complete. It addressed psychiatric nursing and psychotherapy specifically. It did not provide a model for the full scope of medical decision-making that NPs would eventually assume. Nursopathic medicine builds on her precedent while extending it to the breadth of contemporary NP practice.

CHAPTER 3:
DEFINING NURSOPATHIC MEDICINE

Multiple Choice Answers

1. **B – A conceptual framework explaining how NPs practice medicine through advanced nursing**

   Rationale: Nursopathic medicine is "a conceptual framework explaining how NPs practice medicine through advanced nursing". Not new licensure (A), theory replacement (C), or medical specialty (D). Emphasizes it's theoretical explanation of existing practice.

2. **B – The practice domain of diagnosing, treating, and managing disease**

   Rationale: Medicine is "the practice domain of diagnosing, treating, and managing disease through biomedical knowledge". A field of knowledge and practice, not exclusive physician property (A), only allopathic (C), or only hospitals (D).

3. **C – Nurse practitioner practice at the APRN level**

   Rationale: Explicitly stated: applies "specifically to nurse practitioner practice at the advanced practice registered nurse level". Not all nursing (A), only psychiatric (B), or students/educators (D).

4. **B – Professional framework, education, ethics, and licensure grounded in nursing**

   Rationale: Distinguished by "professional framework, education, ethics, and licensure grounded in nursing". Not different diagnostic criteria (A), inability to prescribe (C), or no distinction (D). The professional lens differs fundamentally.

5. **B – Medicine as a practice domain vs. "the practice of medicine" as legal terminology**

   Rationale: The chapter carefully distinguishes "medicine as a practice domain" (field of knowledge/activities) versus "the practice of medicine" as legal/regulatory terminology specific to physicians in state medical practice acts.

6. **B – Allopathic (MD), osteopathic (DO), and nursopathic (NP)**

   Rationale: Medicine as practice domain can be approached through allopathic (MD), osteopathic (DO), and nursopathic (NP) frameworks. Not only allopathic (A), any profession (C), or only medical degrees (D). Each brings distinct values.

7. **B – Educational foundation, epistemological grounding, ethical framework, and professional identity**

   Rationale: What makes it nursing: "educational foundation, epistemological grounding, ethical framework, and professional identity". Not supervision (A), limited scope (C), or nothing (D). Professional framework makes it nursing, not tasks.

8. **B – Integration of nursing identity + medicine + autonomous practice**

   Rationale: Represents "integration of nursing identity + medicine + autonomous practice", not hybridization/blurring (A), abandonment (C), or temporary phase (D). Integration means combining while maintaining distinct identity.

9. **B – Clarity and honesty about what NPs actually do**

   Rationale: Using "medicine" is necessary for "clarity and honesty about what NPs actually do", not legal protection (A), competition (C), or marketing (D). Avoiding the term would obscure NP activities.

10. **C – Nursing licensure (APRN)**

Rationale: "Authority to diagnose and prescribe derives from nursing licensure (advanced practice registered nurse)". Not physician delegation (A), medical licensure (B), or hospital privileges (D). Crucial to understanding autonomous authority within nursing.

Case-Based Application - Suggested Answers

Case Scenario 1:

Question 1: James could explain: "I'm practicing nursopathic medicine, engaging in the practice domain of medicine but AS A NURSE PRACTITIONER through a nursing framework. My education was in nursing programs with nursing's patient-centered approach. I'm licensed as an APRN, accountable to nursing boards, guided by nursing ethics. The ACTIVITIES may look similar to a physician's, but the FRAMEWORK is distinctly nursing."

Question 2: Elements making it distinctly nursing: (a) Education through nursing programs with patient-centered orientation, (b) Professional licensure through nursing (APRN), (c) Epistemological approach emphasizing patient context and relationships, (d) Ethical framework grounded in nursing values, (e) Professional identity as a nurse integrating medical knowledge within nursing scope.

Question 3: While treating the same patient, his practice differs in: (a) Educational preparation (nursing vs. medical school), (b) Professional lens (nursing's holistic approach vs. biomedical focus), (c) Regulatory accountability (nursing boards vs. medical boards), (d) Ethical framework (nursing ethics vs. medical ethics), (e) Professional identity and values. Distinction is in professional framework, not clinical activities.

Case Scenario 2:

Question 1: This reflects the conceptual confusion nursopathic medicine addresses: the false dichotomy between "medicine OR nursing" when NP practice involves medicine THROUGH nursing. The framing assumes these are mutually exclusive, revealing lack of theoretical framework.

Question 2: The correct answer is: "BOTH, we practice medicine through nursing. We engage in the practice domain of medicine but as nurse practitioners through nursing professional framework. This is nursopathic medicine."

Question 3: It's a false dichotomy because it assumes medicine and nursing are mutually exclusive when contemporary NP practice demonstrates integration. The question confuses: (a) Medicine as practice domain vs. "practice of medicine" as legal term, (b) Professional activities vs. professional identity, (c) Task performance vs. professional framework.

True/False Answers

1. **FALSE** - "Not a claim of new licensure, title, or statutory authority, but a theory intended to clarify existing clinical realities."
2. **FALSE** - Medicine as practice domain can be approached through multiple professional frameworks, not exclusive to physicians.
3. **TRUE** - Explicitly stated: "The answer lies in professional framework, not task performance."
4. **FALSE** - Applies only to NP practice at APRN level, not all nursing levels.
5. **TRUE** - Authority derives from nursing licensure (APRN), not medical licensure, fundamental to autonomous practice within nursing.

CHAPTER 4:
METHODS OF CLINICAL REASONING IN NURSOPATHIC MEDICINE

Multiple Choice Answers

1. **B – The five practice domains of the nursopathic medicine model**

   Rationale: The five reasoning methods correspond to and animate the five practice domains of nursopathic medicine. Acute Reasoning corresponds to Acute Care (Chapter 8), Longitudinal Reasoning to Chronic Care (Chapter 9), Anticipatory Reasoning to Preventative Care (Chapter 10), Interdisciplinary Reasoning to Interdisciplinary Care (Chapter 11), and Specialty Lens Reasoning to Specialty Care (Chapter 12). They are not the nursing process, Bloom's taxonomy, or stages of professional formation.

2. **C – What is happening right now, and what must I do?**

   Rationale: Acute Reasoning asks: "What is happening right now, and what must I do?" It is the cognitive mode activated when time is compressed, information is incomplete, and the cost of inaction may be higher than the cost of a provisional decision. The other options describe Longitudinal Reasoning (A), Anticipatory Reasoning (B), and Specialty Lens Reasoning (D).

3. **B – Holds diagnoses as evolving hypotheses refined across repeated encounters**

   Rationale: Longitudinal Reasoning holds diagnoses as working hypotheses subject to revision across repeated encounters — building and refining a dynamic mental model of the patient over time. It is not setting-specific, does not require physician oversight, and does not eliminate Acute Reasoning, which remains active at every encounter regardless of setting.

4. **C – Forward-looking clinical judgment that identifies and acts on foreseeable risks before they manifest**

   Rationale: Anticipatory Reasoning is forward-looking clinical judgment that identifies foreseeable risks and acts on them before they manifest as crises. It is grounded in epidemiology, risk stratification, and prevention evidence — not reactive to presenting symptoms, not limited to protocol-driven checklists, and not exclusive to wellness visits. It applies wherever risk exists.

5. **B – Interdisciplinary Reasoning produces purposeful clinical collaboration; dependency produces deference regardless of clinical indication**

   Rationale: Interdisciplinary Reasoning produces purposeful, clinically indicated collaboration with clear accountability retained by the NP. Dependency is its opposite — reflexive deference driven by regulatory structure or institutional hierarchy rather than clinical indication. Recognizing the limits of scope and initiating a referral is an expression of autonomous practice, not a failure of it.

6. **B – Operates across the entire SOAP note as a pervasive filter, rather than being localized to specific sections**

   Rationale: Specialty Lens Reasoning is the only one of the five methods that does not localize to a specific section of the SOAP note. It operates as a pervasive filter across the entire encounter — shaping what the clinician asks in the Subjective, what data they gather in the Objective, how they frame the differential in the Assessment, and which interventions appear in the Plan.

7. **B – Specialty Lens Reasoning—each practitioner's training equips them with a different primary observational instrument**

   Rationale: The PMHNP's Objective section will center on a Mental Status Examination. The FNP's Objective section will center on a physical examination. Both are correct for their specialty. The difference is not thoroughness — it is that their training equips each clinician with different primary observational instruments. That is Specialty Lens Reasoning: the lens shapes what the clinician looks for and measures.

8. **C – Acute, Longitudinal, Anticipatory, and Interdisciplinary Reasoning—filtered by Specialty Lens Reasoning**

   Rationale: The Assessment section is where all five reasoning methods converge. Acute Reasoning names the working diagnosis. Longitudinal Reasoning asks whether it holds across prior visits. Anticipatory Reasoning stratifies risk. Interdisciplinary Reasoning determines whether this exceeds scope. All of this is filtered by Specialty Lens Reasoning throughout.

9. **B – Interdisciplinary Reasoning—scope boundary recognition as an expression of professional responsibility**

   Rationale: Recognizing when a presentation exceeds one's own scope and initiating appropriate referral is Interdisciplinary Reasoning — not a failure of autonomous practice but one of its clearest expressions. Autonomous practice includes the professional responsibility to accurately assess the limits of one's own competence and engage other disciplines when those limits are reached.

10. **B – It provides a common structure through which all five reasoning methods operate within a single clinical encounter**

    Rationale: The SOAP note is called a "shared clinical language" because it provides the common structure — Subjective, Objective, Assessment, Plan — through which all five reasoning methods operate within a single encounter. It is not merely a billing format, is not required by all state boards, and does not replace documentation of reasoning — it is where that reasoning becomes visible.

Case-Based Application - Suggested Responses

Case Scenario 1 – Alicia and Marcus (Bipolar II, Telehealth)

Which reasoning methods are active and what is each detecting?

Specialty Lens Reasoning activates immediately: in a bipolar II patient, decreased sleep with elevated mood and increased goal-directed activity is a recognized pattern for hypomania, and lamotrigine discontinuation is clinically significant. Acute Reasoning evaluates whether this is a current hypomanic or mixed episode requiring urgent intervention – including safety assessment. Longitudinal Reasoning asks whether this pattern has appeared before, what preceded prior episodes, and how this trajectory compares to his baseline. Anticipatory Reasoning identifies the risk of full manic or mixed episode, impaired judgment, financial harm, and relapse following abrupt medication discontinuation. Interdisciplinary Reasoning evaluates whether this requires escalation to inpatient or intensive outpatient level of care.

Walk through the SOAP note – what does Specialty Lens shape in Subjective? What does Longitudinal Reasoning contribute to Assessment?

In the Subjective, the PMHNP's Specialty Lens directs attention to sleep duration, energy, speech, goal-directed activity, and the patient's own assessment of his mood state – all elements of a hypomanic screening. A generalist lens might not have flagged "sleeping 4 hours and feeling great" as clinically significant. In the Assessment, Longitudinal Reasoning asks: has Marcus had prior hypomanic episodes? What is his typical baseline sleep? Has he stopped lamotrigine before and what happened? The Assessment should note "possible hypomanic episode in context of abrupt lamotrigine discontinuation" with the longitudinal trajectory informing severity and urgency.

How does Acute Reasoning apply in an outpatient telehealth follow-up?

Acute Reasoning is not defined by the setting — it is defined by the cognitive question: what is happening right now, and does it require immediate action? A patient with possible hypomania, impaired sleep, three concurrent projects, and recent medication discontinuation presents real acute risk. Alicia must assess for safety (impulsive behavior, financial decisions, driving), determine whether the current episode requires immediate intervention beyond medication restart, and decide whether the presentation warrants a higher level of care than outpatient telehealth.

What Anticipatory Reasoning should Alicia document in the Plan?

Anticipatory Reasoning in the Plan should address: the risk of escalation to a full hypomanic or mixed episode if lamotrigine is not restarted; the risk of impulsive financial or behavioral decisions during the current elevated period; the importance of sleep as both a symptom marker and a stabilizing intervention; and the plan for follow-up frequency if lamotrigine is restarted and monitoring for tolerability and mood trajectory.

Is Interdisciplinary Reasoning indicated?

Yes. If Alicia determines this meets criteria for hypomania with significant functional impairment or safety risk, she should consider whether this warrants a psychiatry consult (if she is operating outside her usual scope) or intensive outpatient referral. If this is within her PMHNP scope, the Interdisciplinary Reasoning is coordination: ensuring Marcus has a safety support person, communicating with his primary care provider regarding the medication change, and monitoring for emerging medical contributors to the presentation.

Case Scenario 2 – James and Elena (51-year-old Wellness)

Map all five reasoning methods onto James's initial assessment.

Acute Reasoning: BP 138/86 at a wellness visit – is this white coat elevation or sustained hypertension requiring today's intervention? Longitudinal Reasoning: this is a new patient, so James must establish a baseline – what has her BP trended, and how do her symptoms (night sweats, irregular periods, forgetfulness) fit a developing trajectory? Anticipatory Reasoning: clustering risk factors – smoking history, family history of breast and heart disease, perimenopausal symptoms, borderline BP, cognitive changes – identify multiple foreseeable trajectories requiring stratification today. Interdisciplinary Reasoning: this patient may need cardiology (BP, cardiac risk), gynecology or women's health (perimenopausal evaluation), and possibly psychiatry or neurology (cognitive symptoms, anxiety). Specialty Lens Reasoning: as an FNP, James filters everything through a whole-person primary care lens – organizing competing risks, coordinating across systems, thinking about the patient across the lifespan.

How does James's FNP Specialty Lens differ from a PMHNP or women's health NP?

James's FNP lens organizes all five clusters simultaneously – cardiovascular, metabolic, reproductive, cognitive, psychiatric – within a single primary care framework. A PMHNP seeing the same patient would foreground the anxiety and cognitive symptoms, using the MSE and psychiatric differential as the primary frame, and might refer the physical concerns outward. A women's health NP would center the perimenopausal evaluation – hormone levels, menstrual history, vasomotor symptoms – as the organizing framework. James's lens does not go as deep in any one domain but holds the whole person, which is its clinical strength and its defining specialty.

Write the Assessment section demonstrating three reasoning methods.

Assessment: (1) Hypertension, stage 1 (BP 138/86, new patient – baseline not established; requires repeat measurement and cardiovascular risk stratification – Longitudinal and Anticipatory Reasoning). (2) Perimenopause, symptomatic (night sweats, irregular menses × 8 months; FSH, estradiol indicated; breast cancer screening per family history – Anticipatory Reasoning with Specialty Lens). (3) Cardiovascular risk stratification required (15 pack-year smoking history, family history of heart disease, borderline BP, BMI 28.5 – Anticipatory Reasoning). (4) Cognitive and mood symptoms – anxiety and forgetfulness – require differential including perimenopausal cognitive changes, thyroid dysfunction, depression, and early cognitive impairment (Acute Reasoning flags thyroid as actionable today; Specialty Lens organizes the differential).

What Interdisciplinary Reasoning is required and what interface type for each?

Cardiology: referral if BP confirms Stage 1-2 hypertension with elevated 10-year cardiovascular risk; co-management if she has established cardiac risk requiring specialist input alongside FNP longitudinal management. Women's health or gynecology: referral for formal perimenopausal evaluation and hormone therapy discussion if symptom burden is significant. Psychiatry or behavioral health: coordination for anxiety – James may manage this within FNP scope with SSRIs, or refer if complexity warrants specialist input. Radiology/mammography: coordination for breast cancer screening given family history. The key Interdisciplinary Reasoning decision is which concerns James retains versus refers – maintaining his role as the longitudinal primary care anchor while engaging appropriate specialists.

True/False Answers

1. **FALSE**

   Rationale: The five reasoning methods do not operate sequentially. They operate simultaneously and concurrently throughout the clinical encounter. The clinician moves fluidly among them — all five may be active in the first few minutes of an encounter, each informing the others, with one or another foregrounded depending on what the encounter demands.

2. **TRUE**

   Rationale: Specialty Lens Reasoning is the only method that filters the entire SOAP note rather than localizing to a specific section. It shapes what the clinician attends to in the Subjective, what they measure in the Objective, how they frame the differential in the Assessment, and which interventions appear in the Plan. It is active from the first sentence the patient speaks.

3. **FALSE**

   Rationale: Acute Reasoning is defined by cognitive operations — compressed time, incomplete information, threshold judgment, pattern recognition — not by the setting in which it occurs. A PMHNP in an outpatient telehealth session can engage Acute Reasoning just as readily as an NP in an emergency department. The question "what is happening right now, and what must I do?" applies wherever clinical urgency exists.

4. **TRUE**

   Rationale: Longitudinal Reasoning holds every diagnosis as a working hypothesis subject to revision as new data arrives across repeated encounters. A diagnosis made at visit one is not locked in — it is the beginning of a trajectory that subsequent encounters refine. Goals, targets, and clinical priorities evolve as the patient's life and health circumstances change.

5. **FALSE**

Rationale: Anticipatory Reasoning applies wherever risk exists — which is in every clinical setting. A PMHNP monitoring metabolic effects of antipsychotics is performing Anticipatory Reasoning. An acute care NP implementing fall prevention is performing Anticipatory Reasoning. An oncology NP addressing chemotherapy-induced neuropathy is performing Anticipatory Reasoning. It is not limited to wellness visits or primary care.

CHAPTER 5: EDUCATION AND PROFESSIONAL FORMATION IN NURSOPATHIC MEDICINE

Multiple Choice Answers

1. **B – Professional formation: the structured development of clinical reasoning, ethical responsibility, and autonomous accountability**

   Rationale: Education in nursopathic medicine is understood as professional formation — the structured development of clinical reasoning, ethical responsibility, and autonomous accountability. Skill acquisition and task training describe a narrower conception that does not account for the cognitive and identity development that autonomous practice requires. Certification preparation and physician apprenticeship both miss the nursing-centered, autonomy-building purpose of NP education.

2. **B – The NP leads patient care directly, authoring the diagnosis and treatment plan and holding full clinical accountability for the outcome**

   Rationale: The primary difference between the RN and NP roles is not quantity of knowledge or years of training — it is a different structure of clinical authority. The NP authors the diagnosis, treatment plan, prescriptions, and follow-up trajectory, holding full clinical accountability for outcomes. The RN exercises significant clinical judgment within an established framework; the NP establishes the framework.

3. **B – A different relationship to clinical authority—the capacity to author clinical decisions independently and hold full accountability for their outcomes**

   Rationale: The RN entering an NP program most needs to develop a different relationship to clinical authority — the capacity to author clinical decisions independently and hold full accountability for their outcomes. The cognitive shift is not primarily about more knowledge; it is about a fundamentally different orientation to clinical responsibility. The RN's extensive experience is genuinely valuable, but it does not automatically confer the autonomous authority structure that NP practice requires.

4. **C – The student being required to reason independently, defend clinical judgments, and take accountability for decisions before the preceptor intervenes**

   Rationale: Preceptored experience that builds autonomous reasoning requires the student to reason independently, defend clinical judgments, and be accountable for decisions before the preceptor intervenes. Hours alone, observation alone, or variety of settings alone do not produce formation — the cognitive work of reasoning under accountability is what builds the capacity for autonomous practice.

5. **C – Graduate education and national certification**

   Rationale: Scope of practice is determined by graduate education and national certification. Employment setting does not expand scope. An FNP placed in a cardiology clinic remains an FNP. An AGPCNP covering a pediatric unit does not thereby acquire pediatric scope. Professional and legal accountability follows the NP's certification, not the institutional role they have been given.

6. **C – Create conditions in which the student must reason independently, defend judgments, and take responsibility for clinical decisions**

   Rationale: A genuinely formative preceptor creates conditions in which the student must reason independently, defend judgments, and take responsibility for clinical decisions. Demonstrating correct answers, ensuring efficient hour completion, or providing close supervision for every encounter may be helpful practices but do not constitute formation — they keep the cognitive weight with the preceptor rather than transferring it to the student.

7. **B – Developing recognition of limits, appropriate consultation, and commitment to evidence-based standards as intrinsic professional obligations**

   Rationale: Ethical formation includes developing recognition of the limits of one's own competence, the obligation to consult when presentations exceed expertise, and commitment to evidence-based standards as intrinsic professional obligations. It is not memorization of ethics codes, deference to physicians, or protocol compliance — it is the internalization of ethical responsibility as an expression of autonomous accountability.

8. **B – Practicing outside certification scope regardless of institutional support for the role**

   Rationale: An FNP practicing outside their certification scope is doing so regardless of institutional support, job title, or the complexity of the role. The FNP's scope is defined by graduate education and national certification, not by the specialty of the employment setting. Professional and legal consequences follow the clinician, not the institution that placed them in the role.

9. **B – A professional obligation that sustains the alignment between autonomous authority and the competency that authority demands**

   Rationale: Lifelong learning is a professional obligation that sustains the alignment between autonomous authority and the competency that authority demands. Evidence evolves, guidelines are revised, populations change, and pharmacological options expand. Continuing education is not merely a regulatory requirement — it is the mechanism by which autonomous competence remains current with the clinical responsibilities the NP carries.

10. **B – Developed through structured education, supervised clinical experience, and sustained professional responsibility—and maintained through lifelong learning**

    Rationale: Independence in NP practice is developed through structured education, supervised clinical experience, and sustained professional responsibility — and maintained through lifelong learning and reflective practice. It is not conferred at graduation, granted by employers, or achievable through collaboration with physicians. It is built and sustained through formation.

Case-Based Application - Suggested Answers

Case Scenario 1 – Jennifer, FNP, Orthopedic Position

What is the precise scope question Jennifer must answer, and why doesn't the surgeon's confidence resolve it?

The precise scope question is: does Jennifer's FNP graduate education and national certification include preparation for autonomous management of complex orthopedic conditions and post-surgical complications? The surgeon's confidence in Jennifer's learning capacity is clinically and legally irrelevant to this question. Scope is not determined by demonstrated adaptability, on-the-job learning, or institutional confidence in an individual — it is determined by the graduate program that prepared her and the certification that validates that preparation. If the role regularly requires clinical decisions outside FNP scope, Jennifer bears the professional and legal risk regardless of the employer's assurances.

How does employment setting relate to — and specifically not expand — certification scope?

Employment setting describes where an NP works and what the institution asks them to do. Certification scope describes what the NP is prepared and legally authorized to manage. These are different things and can diverge significantly. An institution can place an FNP in an orthopedic practice, call them an orthopedic NP, and give them a job description that includes complex orthopedic care — but none of that changes the FNP's scope. If Jennifer provides care outside her certification scope, the professional and legal consequences fall on her, not the employer who created the role.

What would a responsible path forward look like?

A responsible path would involve: (1) obtaining formal post-graduate education or fellowship training in orthopedic and musculoskeletal care; (2) exploring whether an orthopedic or musculoskeletal subspecialty certification exists or is applicable to her practice population; (3) clearly defining with the employer which clinical functions fall within FNP scope and which require additional preparation; and (4) implementing a structured onboarding period with mentorship and defined scope boundaries that expand only as preparation is verified. Jennifer should not accept a role that begins with the assumption that she will learn out-of-scope practice on the job.

Case Scenario 2 – Marcus, PMHNP, Continuing Education

How does Marcus's attitude conflict with professional formation as lifelong?

Marcus treats formation as terminal – something completed in graduate school and refined by experience, after which no further structured development is required. The chapter argues the opposite: formation is ongoing because the clinical landscape continues to evolve. The PMHNP who practiced five years ago did not have access to current evidence on long-acting injectables, updated diagnostic criteria, evolving pharmacogenomics, or revised treatment guidelines. Graduate school and experience cannot account for what has changed since they were completed. Formation that stops is formation that begins to erode.

Why is experience alone insufficient, and what does continuing education address that experience cannot?

Experience consolidates and deepens what a clinician already knows. It does not introduce new evidence, identify gaps in current practice, or update clinical frameworks that have been revised since training. A clinician who treats hundreds of patients with the same approach every year is gaining depth within a fixed knowledge base – not expanding it. Continuing education provides systematic exposure to current evidence, updated guidelines, emerging pharmacology, and reflective frameworks that allow the clinician to evaluate whether their established practices remain aligned with best evidence. Experience tells you what you have done; continuing education tells you whether what you have done remains the right thing to do.

What are the ethical implications for Marcus's patients?

Autonomous practice carries full clinical accountability – the NP authors the diagnosis and treatment plan and holds responsibility for the outcome. That accountability includes the obligation to maintain competence at a level that matches the authority being exercised. Marcus's patients are receiving care from a clinician who has decided his preparation is complete and requires no updating. If evidence has changed – if a medication he routinely prescribes now has a black box warning, if a diagnostic approach has been revised, if newer first-line treatments exist – his patients are exposed to the gap between his static knowledge base and current best practice. The ethical obligation of autonomous practice is not only to be competent at the time of graduation but to sustain that competence for the duration of practice.

True/False Answers

1. FALSE

   Rationale: Education in nursopathic medicine is understood as professional formation – the structured development of clinical reasoning, ethical responsibility, autonomous accountability, and professional identity. Skill acquisition and biomedical knowledge are components of that formation, but they do not describe its purpose or scope. Formation produces a clinician who can hold ambiguity, reason through uncertainty, and assume full accountability for clinical decisions.

2. **FALSE**

   Rationale: The RN-to-NP transition is primarily a reorientation of professional identity and clinical authority, not a matter of learning new content. RNs entering NP programs often already possess substantial clinical knowledge. What the transition requires is a fundamentally different relationship to clinical authority — the capacity to author decisions, tolerate diagnostic uncertainty without deferring, and stand behind clinical judgments as the accountable clinician of record.

3. **FALSE**

   Rationale: Employment in a specialty clinic does not expand scope. Scope is determined by graduate education and national certification. An FNP working in a cardiology clinic remains an FNP. If the role requires clinical activities outside that scope, the NP bears the professional and legal risk regardless of the institutional context in which those activities occur.

4. **TRUE**

   Rationale: Scope of practice is determined by the graduate program that prepared the NP and the national certification that validates that preparation. Employment setting, institutional credentialing, and the specialty of the clinical role do not alter, expand, or override the certification-based scope. This is one of the chapter's central practical arguments.

5. **TRUE**

   Rationale: Lifelong learning is a professional obligation grounded in the nature of autonomous practice — not merely a regulatory compliance requirement. Evidence evolves, guidelines are revised, clinical populations change, and pharmacological options expand. The NP who stops learning is one whose clinical authority increasingly exceeds the competency base that authority demands. Continuing education is the mechanism by which that alignment is maintained.

CHAPTER 6:
REGULATORY IMPLICATIONS OF NURSOPATHIC MEDICINE

Multiple Choice Answers

1. **B – Licensure, certification, and statutory authority**

   Rationale: "Current regulatory models define nurse practitioner scope through licensure, certification, and statutory authority." Not employment contracts (A), physician preference (C), or hospital policies (D). These formal mechanisms establish boundaries and accountability.

2. **B – Provide conceptual clarity without requiring statutory changes**

   Rationale: Nursopathic medicine's "regulatory implication is conceptual rather than statutory: it offers a language through which existing autonomy can be understood, taught, and evaluated." Not advocating law changes (A), not eliminating requirements (C), not new categories (D). Provides theoretical explanation for existing authority.

3. **B – Authority aligned with licensure and scope, with direct accountability**

   Rationale: Independent practice means "authority aligned with licensure and scope, holding them directly accountable for care." Not isolation from collaboration (A), not absence of regulation (C), not unlimited practice (D). Autonomy with accountability.

4. **B – Mandated supervisory or collaborative arrangements**

   Rationale: Restrictive environments "condition practice on mandated supervisory or collaborative arrangements, regardless of context or competence." Graduate education (A), certification (C), and continuing education (D) are required in all models. The difference is mandated supervision/collaboration.

5. **B – A clinical necessity, not a regulatory constraint**

   Rationale: "Nursopathic medicine affirms collaboration as a clinical necessity rather than a regulatory constraint." Collaboration happens based on clinical need (B), not regulation (A), is valued (not C), not incompetence (D). Clinical judgment determines collaboration.

6. **B – Conceptual**

   Rationale: "Importantly, nursopathic medicine does not propose new titles, licensure categories, or scope expansions. Its regulatory implication is conceptual rather than statutory." Not seeking statutory changes (A), not primarily financial (C), though has international applications (D). Provides conceptual clarity.

7. **B – Varies by province, similar to U.S. state variation**

   Rationale: "Canada's provincial variation creates a natural experiment in regulatory approaches" paralleling "U.S. state-by-state differences." Not uniform (A), does exist (C), variability ranges from restrictive to autonomous (D). Similar pattern to U.S.

8. **B – New titles, licensure categories, or scope expansions**

   Rationale: "Importantly, nursopathic medicine does not propose new titles, licensure categories, or scope expansions." It DOES propose theoretical framework (A), evidence-based practice (C), and professional accountability (D). Explains existing practice, doesn't seek expansion.

9. **B – It describes functional competencies rather than jurisdiction-specific tasks**

   Rationale: The five-domain model "describes functional competencies transcending jurisdiction-specific tasks," making it "adaptable to diverse international contexts." Not because regulations are identical (A), not US-only (C), not claiming qualification differences (D). Functional organization is universal.

10. **B – Offering a language for consistent interpretation without requiring uniform statutes**

    Rationale: "By offering a nursing-centered language for autonomous practice, nursopathic medicine may support clearer communication" and "reduce ambiguity" without "requiring changes to existing regulatory structures." Not changing laws (A), not eliminating regulation (C), not federal mandates (D). Conceptual clarity aids interpretation.

Case-Based Application - Suggested Answers

Case Scenario 1:

Question 1: Nursopathic medicine provides conceptual clarity by explaining WHAT NPs are (nurse practitioners practicing medicine through nursing framework) and HOW their practice works (five functional domains supported by evidence-based practice). Outcome data shows they CAN practice safely; the framework explains WHY their practice is legitimate nursing—grounded in nursing education, ethics, and professional identity. Addresses the "what is this" question data alone can't answer.

Question 2: Theoretical framework reduces concerns because: (a) Explains the nature of NP practice in understandable terms, (b) Shows NPs aren't "pretending to be doctors" but practicing through distinct professional framework, (c) Demonstrates structure and accountability in practice, (d) Addresses conceptual confusion ("is this nursing or medicine?") that data can't resolve, (e) Provides language for understanding role without requiring medical knowledge to evaluate. Theory answers "what is this" while data answers "does it work."

Question 3: Using nursopathic framework: Collaboration ≠ supervision because collaboration is clinical engagement between professionals based on patient need (Interdisciplinary Care domain), while supervision implies hierarchical oversight regardless of clinical indication. NPs collaborate autonomously—they determine when consultation enhances care, maintain accountability for decisions, engage as professional equals. The vine metaphor: collaboration neither "too tight" (constricting autonomy) nor "too loose" (fragmenting care). Clinical necessity, not regulatory constraint.

Case Scenario 2:

Question 1: Regulatory structure affects HOW authority is formally recognized and documented, but doesn't determine professional competence or nursing identity. Maria remains equally competent regardless of province. Restrictive regulations create administrative barriers and may limit practice opportunities, but don't change her professional knowledge, judgment, or nursing framework. Competence is educational/professional; regulation is structural.

Question 2: Maria maintains professional autonomy by: (a) Understanding her authority derives from nursing licensure/certification, not regulation alone, (b) Practicing within nursing scope regardless of collaborative agreement requirements, (c) Making autonomous clinical judgments and decisions within scope, (d) Using collaboration appropriately based on clinical need, not just regulatory compliance, (e) Maintaining professional identity as autonomous NP even in restrictive environment. Autonomy is professional stance, not just regulatory status.

Question 3: The chapter suggests regulation affects how autonomy is formally structured but doesn't determine professional identity or competence. Restrictive regulation creates "external constraints" but nursopathic medicine provides "internal professional framework" that persists regardless of regulatory environment. Professional identity (practicing medicine through nursing) remains constant even when regulations vary.

True/False Answers

1. **FALSE** - Nursopathic medicine does NOT advocate for immediate changes. It provides conceptual clarity for existing practice.
2. **FALSE** - Independent authority comes WITH direct accountability, not without it. Alignment of authority and accountability is core.
3. **TRUE** - Explicitly stated: collaboration is "a clinical necessity rather than a regulatory constraint" in nursopathic medicine.
4. **TRUE** - Canadian provincial variation parallels U.S. state-by-state differences in NP regulation.
5. **FALSE** - The model does NOT require uniform statutes. It provides conceptual language that works across diverse regulatory structures.

CHAPTER 7:
THE NURSOPATHIC MEDICINE PRACTICE MODEL

Multiple Choice Answers

1. **B – Five domains**

   Rationale: "The model consists of five domains" representing distinct yet interconnected dimensions of practice. Not three (A), seven (C), or ten (D). Five functional domains with evidence-based practice foundation.

2. **B – Acute Care, Chronic Care, Preventative Care, Interdisciplinary Care, Specialty Care**

   Rationale: The five domains are specifically: "Acute Care, Chronic Care, Preventative Care, Interdisciplinary Care, and Specialty Care." Not nursing process (A), prevention levels (C), or Benner's stages (D). Functional domains, not process steps.

3. **C – Evidence-Based Practice**

   Rationale: "These five domains rest upon a shared foundation of Evidence-Based Practice, affirming that autonomous authority is exercised within established scientific and professional standards." Not collaboration (A), policies (B), or accreditation (D). Evidence-based practice grounds all domains.

4. **B – Roman**

   Rationale: "The visual metaphor employs classical Roman architectural elements" including Corinthian columns. Not Greek (A), Gothic (C), or Modern (D). Roman architecture chosen for symbolism of strength, stability, permanence.

5. **A – Purity, strength, and timeless nature of professional nursing**

   Rationale: White marble "represents the purity, strength, and timeless nature of professional nursing practice." Not cost (B), hospitals (C), or medical authority (D). Symbolizes nursing's enduring professional values.

6. **B – Unity in collaboration, balanced to neither constrict nor fumble care**

   Rationale: The green vine "represents unity in collaboration" with critical balance: "too tight a grip constricts care" while "too loose a hold fumbles care." Not environmental health (A), natural healing (C), or food (D). Profound symbol of balanced interdisciplinary practice.

7. **B – No domain is subordinate, all are equally essential**

   Rationale: "The equal height of all columns emphasizes that no domain is subordinate to another; all are essential to autonomous practice." Not patient equality (A), salary (C), or specialty identity (D). Professional competency must span all domains.

8. **B – Constricts care and limits autonomous judgment**

   Rationale: When "too tight," the vine "constricts care, limiting flexibility and suffocating autonomous judgment." Not providing support (A), not improving outcomes (C), not strengthening (D). Symbolizes excessive control that undermines autonomy.

9. **B – Specific tasks or settings**

   Rationale: "Rather than defining practice by setting or task, the model describes the reasoning processes and responsibilities that characterize autonomous practice in any context." Organized by function (B), not evidence (A), populations (C), or education (D). Emphasizes how NPs think, not where they work.

10. B – Crisis evaluation (Acute), ongoing management (Chronic), relapse prevention (Preventative), consultation with other disciplines (Interdisciplinary), and psychiatric population expertise (Specialty)

Rationale: "In psychiatric practice, Acute Care includes crisis evaluation and stabilization, while Chronic Care reflects ongoing psychopharmacologic and therapeutic management." Same domains, specialty-specific expression. Not different domains (A), not only Specialty (C) or Acute (D). All five apply across specialties.

11. C – Employment setting determines which domains are used most frequently, but all five remain part of their scope and accountability

Rationale: From the Employment Settings section: "The five domains describe what nurse practitioners are educated and certified to do, not necessarily what every employment setting requires them to do daily. Scope of practice is determined by education, certification, and licensure. Not by employment setting." Even in urgent care emphasizing Acute Care, the NP still engages Preventative Care (risk identification), Interdisciplinary Care (consultation when needed), and other domains. Employment shapes workflow emphasis, not scope. Not "do not apply" (A), not "only accountable for Acute" (B), not "reduced scope" (D).

Case-Based Application - Suggested Answers

Case Scenario 1:

Question 1: The architectural metaphor conveys: (a) Structural relationships, columns supporting roof shows interdependence, (b) Permanence and stability. Marble suggests enduring professional framework, (c) Professional dignity, classical architecture evokes gravitas appropriate to autonomous practice, (d) Visual memorability. Easier to recall than list, (e) Symbolic meaning, green vine, equal heights teach concepts lists can't. Architecture communicates relationships and values beyond content listing.

Question 2: Structural interdependence teaches: (a) All domains necessary, removing any column collapses the structure, (b) Mutual support. Domains reinforce each other in practice, (c) Unified framework, five domains combine to form single professional model (the roof), (d) Balance required. Equal heights show no hierarchy, (e) Foundation matters, all rest on evidence-based practice. List shows parts; architecture shows how parts relate and function together.

Question 3: Visual model aids professional identity by: (a) Providing memorable representation of "what NPs do," (b) Showing structure and coherence of practice, (c) Symbolizing professional values (marble = strength, vine = collaboration), (d) Creating shared language for the profession, (e) Conveying complexity and sophistication of autonomous practice. Students see themselves building something substantial and enduring.

Case Scenario 2:

Question 1: Using equal-height columns: "Yes, the five-domain model applies to urgent care practice. Equal-height columns mean all five domains remain part of your scope and accountability regardless of employment setting. The employment setting determines workflow emphasis, not competency requirements or scope. Even though Acute Care dominates your daily work, you still engage the other domains."

Question 2: Concrete examples in urgent care: (a) Acute Care, episodic problem evaluation (your primary activity), (b) Chronic Care. Recognizing poorly controlled diabetes in a patient presenting for wound care, providing interim guidance and facilitating PCP follow-up, (c) Preventative Care, identifying hypertension during a URI visit, providing counseling and initiating appropriate screening or referral, (d) Interdisciplinary Care. Consulting when presentations exceed scope or warrant specialty input (chest pain requiring cardiology evaluation), (e) Specialty Care, applying population-specific knowledge (pediatric vs. geriatric presentations differ). All five domains operate even when Acute dominates.

Question 3: Employment setting vs. scope distinction: (a) Scope is determined by education, certification, and licensure, not by where you work, (b) Employment setting determines which domains you use most frequently, not which domains are part of your scope, (c) You cannot claim "I only do acute care" to avoid accountability for recognizing chronic disease gaps or making appropriate referrals, (d) An urgent care NP encountering uncontrolled diabetes must address it appropriately (assess acute presentation, recognize chronic gap, provide interim guidance, facilitate follow-up). Employment doesn't exempt you from comprehensive assessment, (e) Accountability matters because you remain responsible for competency across all five domains even if your daily workflow emphasizes one. This prevents fragmented care and maintains professional standards.

True/False Answers

1. **FALSE** - The model consists of five domains, not three.
2. **TRUE** - Explicitly stated: "All five domains rest on Evidence-Based Practice foundation."
3. **TRUE** - The green vine represents "unity in collaboration, balanced to neither constrict nor fumble care."
4. **FALSE** - When too tight, vine constricts care and limits autonomy. Appropriate structure requires balance.
5. **FALSE** - Model is organized by functional domains (Acute, Chronic, etc.), not specific tasks or settings. Function over task.

CHAPTER 8:
ACUTE CARE

Multiple Choice Answers

1. **B – Assumption of responsibility under conditions of uncertainty**

   Rationale: Acute Care is "defined by assumption of responsibility for clinical outcomes under conditions of uncertainty". Not by setting (A), not requiring supervision (C), and not limited to simple cases (D). The defining feature is taking responsibility when information is incomplete and time is limited.

2. **B – Episodic assessment, diagnostic reasoning, and timely intervention for time-sensitive conditions**

   Rationale: Acute Care "encompasses the capacity to rapidly assess, synthesize clinical information, establish working diagnoses, and initiate timely interventions in response to emergent, unstable, or time-sensitive conditions." Not only emergencies (A), not wellness (C), not only scheduled procedures (D).

3. **B – Incomplete data requiring management of uncertainty**

   Rationale: "Acute clinical environments compress time, increase risk, and limit information. In this context, decisions are often made with incomplete data." Not complete information (A), not physician direction (C), not unlimited time (D). Managing uncertainty responsibly is central to acute care.

4. **B – Rapidly synthesize clinical information despite time constraints**

   Rationale: Pattern recognition allows NPs to "rapidly assess, synthesize clinical information, establish working diagnoses, and initiate timely interventions" despite time pressure. Not avoiding reasoning (A), not delaying (C), not transferring all care (D). Essential cognitive skill for acute situations.

5. **B – Risk of action vs. inaction, escalation vs. stabilization**

   Rationale: "A central feature of acute decision-making is the determination of thresholds for intervention. Nurse practitioners must continuously evaluate the risk of action versus inaction, escalation versus stabilization." Not billing (A), not only preferences (C), not insurance (D). Clinical risk assessment.

6. **B – Clear articulation of assessment, decision pathways, and response to change**

   Rationale: "Autonomous acute decision-making carries explicit accountability for patient outcomes. Documentation serves not only legal or institutional purposes, but also reflects professional reasoning." Not countersignature (A), not transferring responsibility (C), not avoiding documentation (D).

7. **B – Acute exacerbations occur in patients with ongoing conditions**

   Rationale: "Acute Care does not exist in isolation. It intersects with Chronic Care when acute exacerbations occur in patients with ongoing conditions." Not separate (A), not setting-specific (C), not regulatory (D). Domains integrate in practice.

8. **B – Wherever patient stability can change rapidly**

   Rationale: "Acute clinical decision-making is not confined to emergency departments or inpatient units. It occurs wherever patient stability can change rapidly, including outpatient clinics, psychiatric settings, and specialty practices." Not ED-only (A), not hospital-only (C), not time-limited (D).

9. **B – Acute Care, crisis evaluation and stabilization**

   Rationale: A PMHNP performing "crisis evaluation, risk stratification for suicide or violence, and initiation of stabilization strategies in acute psychiatric presentations" is demonstrating Acute Care domain. Not only Chronic (A), not only Preventative (C), not only Specialty (D). Crisis = acute.

10. **B – Recognize limits and initiate appropriate escalation when warranted**

    Rationale: "The nurse practitioner's authority lies in the capacity to manage uncertainty responsibly" which includes "the responsibility to recognize limits and to initiate appropriate escalation when warranted." Not always independent (A), not never consulting (C), not avoiding difficult cases (D). Autonomous practice includes knowing when to escalate.

Case-Based Application - Suggested Answers

Case Scenario 1:

Question 1: Maria demonstrates autonomous Acute Care by: (a) Immediate pattern recognition (chest pressure + risk factors = ACS), (b) Initiating interventions independently (aspirin, nitroglycerin, oxygen, IV access), (c) Obtaining 12-lead EKG and interpreting findings (STEMI), (d) Activating emergency response (calling EMS, cath lab), (e) Making time-critical decisions without waiting for physician approval, (f) Documenting reasoning and interventions with accountability. She exercises independent clinical authority under extreme time pressure.

Question 2: Maria balances immediate intervention with escalation by: (a) Recognizing this exceeds clinic capabilities and requires emergent cardiology intervention, (b) Starting treatment immediately (aspirin, nitro, O2) while arranging transfer, (c) Not delaying interventions to consult but acting within scope, (d) Activating cath lab so team is ready on arrival, (e) Providing seamless handoff to EMS and hospital, (f) Understanding her scope includes recognizing need for specialist care. Autonomous doesn't mean managing everything independently—means making independent judgment about what's needed.

Question 3: Delaying for "more information" or "calling collaborating physician" could have resulted in: (a) Delayed aspirin/antiplatelet therapy (increasing MI size, (b) Delayed cath lab activation) missing critical time window, (c) Larger infarct, more myocardial damage, (d) Increased risk of complications/death, (e) Moral and legal liability for preventable harm. In acute situations with clear emergent presentations, waiting for permission when authority exists is negligence. Autonomous practice means acting when action is indicated.

Case Scenario 2:

Question 1: David's differential demonstrates comprehensive acute reasoning by considering: (a) Bupropion-induced psychosis (medication-related, temporal correlation), (b) Underlying bipolar disorder now unmasked (psychiatric), (c) Medical causes. Infection, metabolic derangement (organic), (d) Substance intoxication despite negative admission tox screen, (e) Rapid cycling or mixed episode (psychiatric). He systematically considers medication, psychiatric, and medical causes, holistic differential for acute mental status change.

Question 2: David balances safety with uncertainty by: (a) Ensuring immediate safety (constant observation, secured environment), (b) Treating acute symptoms (olanzapine, lorazepam for agitation/psychosis), (c) Simultaneously investigating causes (holding bupropion, ordering labs, requesting medical consult), (d) Not waiting for definitive diagnosis to address safety, (e) Reassessing frequently as information emerges. Safety takes priority while diagnostic workup proceeds—managing uncertainty without paralysis.

Question 3: Holding bupropion demonstrates autonomous judgment because: (a) Recognizes temporal relationship (psychosis appeared after bupropion start), (b) Acts on clinical reasoning without needing psychiatrist approval, (c) Applies pharmacologic knowledge (bupropion can cause psychosis), (d) Takes responsibility for reversing potentially causative medication, (e) Makes independent prescribing decision. This is autonomous prescriptive authority based on clinical assessment—not following preset protocols or waiting for approval.

True/False Answers

1. **FALSE** - Acute Care is defined by "assumption of responsibility under conditions of uncertainty", function, not setting.
2. **FALSE** - Decisions are "often made with incomplete data and must balance immediacy against safety." Managing uncertainty is central.
3. **TRUE** - Pattern recognition is explicitly described as essential reasoning process in acute contexts for rapid synthesis.
4. **TRUE** - "The nurse practitioner's authority lies in the capacity to manage uncertainty responsibly" which includes "responsibility to recognize limits and initiate appropriate escalation."
5. **FALSE** - Acute Care integrates with Interdisciplinary Care when consultation/referral needed. Collaboration enhances acute care.

CHAPTER 9:
CHRONIC CARE

Multiple Choice Answers

1. **B – Sustained responsibility for monitoring and management over time**

   Rationale: Chronic Care is "defined by sustained responsibility for patient care over time" encompassing "ongoing assessment, monitoring, adjustment, and evaluation of treatment plans across the trajectory of illness or wellness." Not episodic (A), not acute (C), not only screening (D).

2. **B – Unfolds across repeated encounters, recognizing patterns over time**

   Rationale: "Longitudinal clinical reasoning unfolds across repeated encounters rather than discrete moments. Nurse practitioners must recognize patterns, trends, and deviations that emerge only through sustained observation." Not single encounters (A), not unnecessary (C), not requiring referral (D). Time reveals what single visits cannot.

3. **B – Continuous monitoring of therapeutic effectiveness and safety**

   Rationale: "A defining feature of Chronic Care is continuous monitoring of therapeutic effectiveness and safety. Nurse practitioners must determine when treatment is effective, when modification is required, and when alternative strategies should be considered." Not episodic (A), not crisis (C), not single diagnosis (D).

4. **B – Functional status, quality of life, and risk mitigation**

   Rationale: "Outcome evaluation extends beyond symptom control to include functional status, quality of life, and risk mitigation." Not only labs (A), not only satisfaction (C), not only adherence (D). Holistic outcomes assessment.

5. **B – Deliberate reflection on whether clinical goals are being met**

   Rationale: "Longitudinal accountability requires deliberate reflection on whether clinical goals are being met and whether care remains aligned with patient needs and evidence-based standards." Not frequency (A), not automatic referral (C), not rigidity (D). Active ongoing evaluation.

6. **B – An active process requiring intentional communication and coordination**

   Rationale: "Continuity is an active process rather than a passive outcome. It involves intentional communication, coordination, and clinical oversight to preserve coherence in care delivery despite system fragmentation." Not passive (A), not automatic (C), not unnecessary (D). Requires deliberate effort.

7. **B – Serves as both clinical insight source and foundation for shared decision-making**

   Rationale: "The therapeutic relationship serves as both a source of clinical insight and a foundation for shared decision-making" in longitudinal care. Not a barrier (A), not to be avoided (C), not only mental health (D). Essential to Chronic Care.

   8. B - May require revision, authority includes ability to reassess and recalibrate

   Rationale: "As conditions evolve, initial diagnoses and management strategies may require revision. The nurse practitioner's authority lies in the ability to reassess, recalibrate, and redirect care in response to change." Not unchangeable (A), not deferring (C), not permanent (D). Adaptation is essential.

9. **B – Longitudinal reasoning, continuity, and sustained accountability**

   Rationale: Managing multiple chronic conditions for five years demonstrates "longitudinal reasoning, continuity, and sustained accountability", core features of Chronic Care domain. Not fragmented (A), not inability to refer (C), not scope creep (D). Sustained comprehensive care.

10. **B – Across all NP specialties regardless of setting or population**

    Rationale: "Chronic Care occurs across all nurse practitioner specialties, regardless of setting or population. Whether managing chronic disease, psychiatric conditions, recovery trajectories, or specialty-specific care, nurse practitioners exercise autonomous authority through sustained engagement." Not only primary care (A), not only elderly (C), not only outpatient (D). Universal domain.

Case-Based Application - Suggested Answers

Case Scenario 1:

Question 1: Jennifer's 5-year perspective differs by: (a) Recognizing gradual progression (prediabetes → diabetes, cognitive changes over time), (b) Seeing patterns across multiple visits (medication responses, adherence issues, life circumstances), (c) Adjusting goals as conditions evolve (post-TIA risk reduction changes everything), (d) Building trust enabling difficult conversations (driving, cognition), (e) Understanding accumulated impact of decisions (multiple chronic conditions requiring coordinated management). Each visit in isolation misses trajectory and accumulated context.

Question 2: Without sustained relationship and continuity: (a) Subtle cognitive decline might be missed or dismissed, (b) Post-TIA care wouldn't connect to pre-TIA prevention opportunities, (c) Trust for difficult conversations wouldn't exist, (d) Medication adjustments wouldn't reflect response patterns over time, (e) Patient would experience fragmented care with repeated explanations. Longitudinal accountability catches what episodic care misses.

Question 3: Longitudinal accountability shaped decisions by: (a) Intensifying prevention after TIA (accountable for missed prevention opportunities), (b) Adjusting diabetes targets based on TIA risk (evidence-based adaptation to changed circumstances), (c) Addressing cognition proactively rather than waiting for crisis, (d) Coordinating multiple specialists while maintaining overall responsibility, (e) Balancing aggressive treatment with quality of life over time. Sustained responsibility drives more thoughtful, individualized care.

Case Scenario 2:

Question 1: Longitudinal reasoning adds: (a) Pattern recognition across multiple encounters (medication responses, adherence patterns, lifestyle factors), (b) Understanding patient's lived experience with condition over time, (c) Trajectory analysis—is patient improving, stable, or declining?, (d) Relationship-based insights patients share only with sustained trust, (e) Accountability for cumulative outcomes, not just today's decision. Single-encounter reasoning optimizes one visit; longitudinal reasoning optimizes the patient's life trajectory.

Question 2: Example requiring longitudinal perspective: Patient has tried three antihypertensives with side effects. Longitudinal reasoning reveals: (a) Pattern (all caused same side effect (dizziness), (b) Life context) patient lives alone, falls are high risk, (c) Previous discussions about medication preferences, (d) Current blood pressure compared to trend over 2 years, (e) Whether goals need adjustment based on functional priorities. Single encounter sees "blood pressure elevated today"; longitudinal sees "pattern of medication intolerance requiring different strategy."

Question 3: Continuity is "active process" because: (a) Systems fragment care by default, requires effort to maintain coherence, (b) Must intentionally communicate across transitions (hospital, specialists, ER), (c) Requires tracking patient across time despite gaps in visits, (d) Must synthesize information from multiple sources into unified plan, (e) EMRs don't create continuity. Just information access. Continuity requires deliberate effort, not just having access to records.

True/False Answers

1. **FALSE** - Chronic Care is characterized by "sustained responsibility for monitoring and management over time," not episodic encounters.
2. **TRUE** - "Patterns, trends, and deviations emerge only through sustained observation" across time, defining feature of longitudinal reasoning.
3. **FALSE** - Continuity is "an active process rather than passive outcome" requiring "intentional communication and coordination"—not automatic.
4. **TRUE** - Explicitly stated: outcome evaluation "extends beyond symptom control to include functional status, quality of life, and risk mitigation."
5. **FALSE** - Chronic Care "occurs across all nurse practitioner specialties, regardless of setting or population." Not limited to primary care.

CHAPTER 10:
PREVENTATIVE CARE

Multiple Choice Answers

1. **B – A professional obligation embedded within all clinical decision-making**

   Rationale: Preventative Care is "understood not as a discrete service line, but as a professional obligation embedded within all clinical decision-making." Not separate service (A), not only wellness visits (C), not same as public health (D). Integrated throughout practice.

2. **B – Recognizing emerging risks before they manifest as acute conditions**

   Rationale: "Anticipatory clinical reasoning, the capacity to recognize emerging risks before they manifest as acute or irreversible conditions." Not reactive (A), not crisis (C), not referral (D). Forward-looking, proactive reasoning.

3. **B – The intensity and timing of preventive actions**

   Rationale: "Risk stratification guides the intensity and timing of preventive actions." Not billing (A), not medication costs (C), not scheduling (D). Clinical decision-making about prevention strategies.

4. **C – Waiting for symptoms to appear**

   Rationale: Prevention includes "screening, counseling, anticipatory guidance, and interventions designed to reduce morbidity and prevent avoidable complications". NOT waiting for symptoms (C). Prevention is proactive by definition. Includes A, B, D.

5. **B – Treatment-related adverse effects**

   Rationale: "Harm mitigation extends to the prevention of treatment-related adverse effects. Nurse practitioners practicing autonomously must balance therapeutic benefit with potential risk." Not only liability (A), not only complaints (C), not only regulatory (D). Includes iatrogenic prevention.

6. **B – Across acute, chronic, specialty, and procedural environments**

   Rationale: "Preventative Care is not confined to primary care or wellness settings. It occurs across acute, chronic, specialty, and procedural environments." Not only primary care (A), not only wellness (C), not only healthy patients (D). Universal application.

   7. B - Preventative Care, anticipatory harm mitigation

   Rationale: Monitoring metabolic risks from antipsychotics is "prevention of treatment-related adverse effects". Preventative Care domain. Not Acute (A), not only Chronic (C), not overstepping (D). Anticipating and preventing iatrogenic harm.

8. **B – Not treated as adjunct but as core clinical responsibility**

   Rationale: "By framing prevention as a function of clinical reasoning rather than a checklist of services, this domain remains applicable across populations, practice settings, and evolving standards of care." Not adjunct (A), not optional (C), not only healthy (D). Core responsibility.

9. **B – Identifying and addressing risks before problems occur**

   Rationale: Anticipatory guidance involves "forward-looking approach" to "recognize emerging risks before they manifest" and "intervene proactively." Not less important (A), not requiring special training (C), not impossible to document (D). Proactive vs. reactive.

10. **B – Preventative Care integrated into acute care setting**

    Rationale: Fall prevention in hospitalized elder demonstrates "Preventative Care is not confined to primary care or wellness settings. It occurs across acute, chronic, specialty, and procedural environments." Not outside scope (A), not only assistant tasks (C), not PT (D). Prevention integrated everywhere.

Case-Based Application - Suggested Answers

Case Scenario 1:

Question 1: Comprehensive risk stratification differs by: (a) Recognizing clustering/synergy of risks (prediabetes + hypertension + dyslipidemia + family history = high CV risk), (b) Identifying connections (sleep apnea worsens hypertension, anxiety affects adherence), (c) Prioritizing intervention targets (which risks most urgent?), (d) Addressing root causes (stress, sedentary lifestyle) not just symptoms, (e) Creating integrated prevention plan rather than treating 6 separate problems. Isolation misses the big picture—patient is one person with interconnected risks.

Question 2: Prevention operates across domains by: (a) Cardiovascular prevention (statin, aspirin consideration, lifestyle), (b) Metabolic prevention (DPP referral, preventing diabetes), (c) Sleep disorder prevention (treating OSA prevents CV/metabolic complications), (d) Mental health prevention (preventing anxiety/depression worsening that undermines other efforts), (e) Future frailty prevention (establishing exercise now). All domains addressed simultaneously because they interact.

Question 3: This is "anticipatory reasoning" not just "screening" because: (a) Goes beyond checking boxes on prevention checklist, (b) Synthesizes multiple data points into risk assessment, (c) Individualizes based on patient context (family history changes risk calculation), (d) Prioritizes among competing prevention targets, (e) Anticipates future trajectories (preventing father's fate—MI at 58). Screening is task completion; anticipatory reasoning is clinical judgment about future risks.

Case Scenario 2:

Question 1: Prevention requires judgment because: (a) Guidelines provide general recommendations, not specific patient orders, (b) Must individualize based on patient risks, values, circumstances, (c) Must prioritize among multiple guideline recommendations (can't do everything), (d) Must balance benefits vs. harms for this patient, (e) Must decide timing, intensity, frequency of interventions. Guidelines inform; judgment determines application to individual.

Question 2: Example of individualization: USPSTF recommends colon cancer screening starting age 45. But patient with strong family history (father diagnosed at 50) should start earlier (age 40 or 10 years before father's diagnosis). Patient with severe comorbidities and limited life expectancy may not benefit from screening. Guidelines set framework; clinical judgment individualizes.

Question 3: Prevention is "core responsibility" because: (a) Autonomous practice includes anticipating and preventing foreseeable harm, (b) Professional accountability extends to prevention, not just treatment, (c) Evidence-based practice includes prevention evidence, (d) Patient safety depends on risk mitigation, (e) Holistic care addresses future health, not just current problems. Task completion meets minimum standards; professional responsibility means thoughtful, individualized prevention.

True/False Answers

1. **FALSE** - Preventative Care is "not as a discrete service line, but as a professional obligation embedded within all clinical decision-making."
2. **TRUE** - Anticipatory reasoning is defined as "recognizing emerging risks before they manifest as acute or irreversible conditions."
3. **FALSE** - "Preventative Care is not confined to primary care or wellness settings. It occurs across acute, chronic, specialty, and procedural environments."
4. **TRUE** - Monitoring metabolic effects from antipsychotics is explicitly given as example of Preventative Care—iatrogenic harm prevention.
5. **FALSE** - "Preventive actions are selected based on evidence, patient context, and clinical judgment rather than rote protocol adherence."

CHAPTER 11:
INTERDISCIPLINARY CARE

Multiple Choice Answers

1. **B – Collaborative engagement across professions while maintaining autonomous clinical authority**

   Rationale: Interdisciplinary Care is "collaborative engagement across professions while maintaining autonomous clinical authority within nursing's scope." Not supervision (A), not replacing autonomy (C), not delegation (D). Collaboration enhances but doesn't replace autonomous practice.

2. **B – Unity in collaboration, balanced to neither constrict nor fumble care**

   Rationale: The green vine "represents unity in collaboration, balanced to neither constrict nor fumble care." Critical visual metaphor for interdisciplinary relationships. Not organic practice (A), not natural healing (C), not hierarchies (D). Symbolizes balanced collaboration.

3. **B – Excessive oversight that constricts care and limits autonomous judgment**

   Rationale: When "too tight," the vine "constricts care, limiting flexibility and suffocating autonomous judgment", represents over-regulation or micromanagement. Not good structure (A), not appropriate (C), not safety (D). Symbolizes harmful over-control.

4. **B – Care fumbled through insufficient coordination and fragmented delivery**

   Rationale: When "too loose," care is "fumbled through insufficient coordination and communication, resulting in fragmented delivery." Not maximum autonomy (A), not true independence (C), not reduced liability (D). Symbolizes inadequate collaboration.

5. **B – Operates alongside autonomous practice**

   Rationale: "Interdisciplinary collaboration operates alongside autonomous practice, not instead of it." Collaboration and autonomy coexist. Not replacement (A), not only regulatory (C), not incompetence (D). Complementary, not contradictory.

6. **B – Autonomous clinical contribution within nursing's professional framework**

   Rationale: NPs contribute "autonomous clinical judgment within nursing's professional framework" to interdisciplinary teams, as professional peers. Not subordination (A), not only tasks (C), not absence of decision-making (D). Professional equality.

7. **B – Is chosen based on clinical need, not hierarchical requirement**

   Rationale: Consultation is "sought based on clinical need rather than hierarchical requirement" unlike supervision which is mandated. Not mandatory (A), not incompetence (C), doesn't transfer accountability (D). Clinical judgment drives consultation.

8. **B – Clear communication while maintaining professional accountability**

   Rationale: Appropriate interdisciplinary engagement requires "clear communication, mutual respect, and shared commitment to patient welfare" while "each professional maintains accountability within their scope." Not physician approval (A), not abandoning judgment (C), not avoiding collaboration (D).

9. **B – Professional relationships require thoughtful calibration**

   Rationale: The vine metaphor teaches that "professional relationships require thoughtful calibration", neither excessive control nor inadequate coordination. Not unnecessary (A), not always more oversight (C), not isolation (D). Balance is key.

10. **B – Professional maturity recognizing when specialist input enhances care**

    Rationale: Consultation demonstrates "professional maturity, recognizing when specialist input enhances care" within context of autonomous practice. Not inability (A), not scope violation (C), not only compliance (D). Sign of sophisticated judgment.

Case-Based Application - Suggested Answers

Case Scenario 1:

Question 1: First hospital: "Vine too tight", co-signature requirements constrain autonomous judgment even for routine care, suggesting distrust and micromanagement. Second hospital: Balanced vine. AGACNPs practice independently with consultation based on clinical need, collaboration as professional peers. First creates bureaucratic barriers; second enables optimal practice.

Question 2: First model consequences: (a) Delays in care requiring signatures, (b) Undermines AGACNP competence and confidence, (c) Creates inefficiency, (d) Signals distrust, (e) May reduce recruitment/retention. Second model consequences: (a) Timely decisions, (b) Professional respect and satisfaction, (c) Appropriate use of specialist expertise when needed, (d) Attracts qualified AGACNPs, (e) Efficient care delivery. Patient care suffers with vine too tight.

Question 3: Second model demonstrates Interdisciplinary Care domain by: (a) AGACNPs maintain autonomous authority and accountability, (b) Consult specialists based on clinical judgment, not mandate, (c) Collaborate as professional peers, not subordinates, (d) Communication flows bidirectionally with mutual respect, (e) Each professional accountable within their scope. This is interdisciplinary practice—collaboration alongside autonomy.

Case Scenario 2:

Question 1: Demonstrates autonomous practice coexisting with collaboration by: (a) Sarah maintains primary responsibility for psychiatric care, (b) She independently identifies need for cardiology consultation, (c) She engages collaboratively but as professional peer, (d) She contributes nursing expertise on psychiatric medications, (e) Shared decision-making respects both specialties, (f) She retains accountability for psychiatric management. Autonomous doesn't mean isolated.

Question 2: This is interdisciplinary engagement not supervision because: (a) Sarah chose to consult based on clinical need, not regulatory requirement, (b) Cardiologist doesn't approve/disapprove Sarah's plan but collaborates, (c) Each maintains accountability in their domain, (d) Expertise is bidirectional—Sarah knows psych meds, cardiologist knows cardiac effects, (e) Professional peers problem-solving together. Consultation ≠ supervision.

Question 3: "Vine too tight": Cardiologist insists on approving all psychiatric medications, or Sarah must get cardiology clearance for routine psychiatric care, unnecessary oversight constraining autonomy. "Vine too loose": No communication between Sarah and cardiology, each makes changes unilaterally without coordination, resulting in medication interactions. Fragmented care. Current scenario: balanced, appropriate consultation maintaining autonomous practice.

True/False Answers

1. **FALSE** - “Interdisciplinary collaboration operates alongside autonomous practice, not instead of it.” Enhances, doesn’t replace.
2. **TRUE** - The vine metaphor explicitly teaches that collaboration requires balance—”neither constrict nor fumble care.”
3. **FALSE** - When “too tight,” vine “constricts care, limiting flexibility and suffocating autonomous judgment”—harmful, not supportive.
4. **TRUE** - Consultation based on clinical judgment “demonstrates professional maturity, recognizing when specialist input enhances care.”
5. **FALSE** - Interdisciplinary engagement maintains accountability—”each professional maintains accountability within their scope of practice.”

CHAPTER 12:
SPECIALTY CARE

Multiple Choice Answers

1. **B – Population- or condition-focused expertise informing advanced practice within defined domains**

   Rationale: Specialty Care is "population- or condition-focused expertise that informs advanced assessment, diagnosis, and management within defined clinical domains." Not employment (A), not experience alone (C), not hospital privileges (D). Defined by education and expertise.

2. **B – The specialty for which formally educated and nationally certified**

   Rationale: "Scope alignment requires that autonomous specialty practice be exercised within the specialty for which the nurse practitioner is formally educated and nationally certified, not simply the setting in which they are employed." Not any specialty (A), not experience-based (C), not employer-determined (D). Education and certification determine scope.

3. **B – Practices as an FNP within FNP scope in that setting**

   Rationale: "A family nurse practitioner employed in a cardiology clinic practices as a family nurse practitioner (applying FNP scope to patients within that setting) not as a cardiology specialist." Not automatic specialist (A), not cardiologist (C), still an NP (D). Employment ≠ scope.

4. **B – Scope is determined by certification, not employment**

   Rationale: "This distinction is critical for several reasons" including "Professional Accountability: Nurse practitioners remain accountable to their certification and licensure scope regardless of employment." Critical principle. Not salary (A), not parking (C), settings matter but don't determine scope (D).

5. **B – Graduate education, national certification, and documented competency in that specialty**

   Rationale: "Legitimate specialty practice within nursopathic medicine occurs when: (1) Formal education exists, (2) Certification is obtained, (3) Supervised transition occurs, (4) Scope remains clear." Not employment only (A), not physician approval (C), not experience alone (D). Formal preparation required.

6. **B – Population- and context-focused**

   Rationale: "Nurse practitioner specialty practice is organized differently: Population-focused rather than organ-system focused (adult-gerontology, pediatric, neonatal, women's health)." Not organ-system like medicine (A), not identical to physician subspecialties (C), not unorganized (D). Distinct nursing approach.

7. **B – Applying specialty medical knowledge through a nursing framework**

   Rationale: Specialty-certified NPs "apply specialty medical knowledge through a nursing framework, maintaining their professional identity while exercising specialized expertise." Not becoming physicians (A), not abandoning nursing (C), not illegal (D). Integration within nursing.

8. **B – Professional obligations in autonomous practice**

   Rationale: "Autonomous practice includes the professional obligation to recognize the limits of one's expertise and to consult or refer when patient needs exceed one's scope." Not incompetence (A), not unnecessary (C), not only for new grads (D). Expression of professional responsibility.

9. **B – Deep familiarity with physiologic, psychological, developmental, or procedural characteristics of specialty populations**

   Rationale: Population-focused expertise involves "deep familiarity with the physiologic, psychological, developmental, or procedural characteristics that distinguish their specialty populations." Not only demographics (A), not marketing (C), not geography (D). Clinical expertise specific to population.

10. **B – An expression of professional responsibility**

    Rationale: "Consultation, collaboration, and recognition of limits... Autonomous practice includes the professional obligation to recognize the limits of one's expertise." Not limitation (A), not incompetence (C), not unnecessary for experienced (D). Demonstrates professional maturity.

Case-Based Application - Suggested Answers

Case Scenario 1:

Question 1: Jennifer should ask: (a) Does this role require FNP scope or orthopedic specialty scope?, (b) What education/training is provided for orthopedic-specific competencies?, (c) Is orthopedic certification required or available?, (d) How will complex orthopedic cases be managed (consultation? referral?), (e) What is the pathway to appropriate certification if needed?, (f) How does liability align with scope (am I covered for specialty-level care with generalist credentials?).

Question 2: Employment doesn't expand scope because: (a) Scope determined by education and certification, not job title, (b) Professional accountability remains to FNP standards regardless of where employed, (c) Licensure and certification boards define scope, not employers, (d) Patient safety depends on practicing within competency boundaries, (e) Legal liability follows certification, not employment. Can't practice beyond education/certification just because employer offers the job.

Question 3: Appropriate preparation: (a) Orthopedic NP fellowship or formal certificate program, (b) Orthopedic specialty certification (if available), (c) Documented supervised clinical experience with orthopedic preceptors, (d) Competency validation in orthopedic assessment, procedures, management, (e) Clear understanding of when to consult orthopedic surgeon. Employment alone doesn't substitute for formal specialty preparation.

Case Scenario 2:

Question 1: Her practice is distinctly nursing because: (a) Education was through nursing programs with nursing's patient-centered orientation, (b) Licensed and accountable as APRN, not physician, (c) Approaches cancer care through nursing lens—holistic, functional outcomes, patient experience, (d) Guided by nursing ethics (advocacy, empowerment, relationships), (e) Professional identity as nurse applying oncology expertise through nursing framework. Activities look medical; framework is nursing.

Question 2: Nursing's population focus (oncology NP cares for cancer patients holistically, physical, psychological, social, family impact) differs from medicine's organ-system focus (medical oncologist treats specific cancer types/organs). Nursing organizes by who is served (population); medicine organizes by what is treated (disease/organ). Different professional lens on same patient.

Question 3: Distinction is professionally important because: (a) Clarifies NPs aren't "junior oncologists" but autonomous nursing specialists, (b) Maintains professional identity within nursing rather than adopting medical identity, (c) Preserves nursing values and approach in specialty practice, (d) Supports appropriate scope boundaries—NP practicing nursing, not medicine in physician-specific sense, (e) Explains to others (patients, colleagues) what specialty NPs are. Prevents identity confusion and role misunderstanding.

True/False Answers

1. **FALSE** - Specialty Care is defined by "population- or condition-focused expertise," not employment setting. Employment doesn't determine scope.
2. **FALSE** - "A family nurse practitioner employed in a cardiology clinic practices as a family nurse practitioner"—not automatic specialist.
3. **TRUE** - "Legitimate specialty practice requires: (1) Graduate-level education, (2) National certification, (3) Supervised transition, (4) Clear scope." Formal preparation required.
4. **FALSE** - Consultation and referral are "professional obligations in autonomous practice", expression of professional responsibility, not incompetence.
5. **TRUE** - "Recognition of limits... Autonomous practice includes the professional obligation to recognize the limits of one's expertise"—expression of responsibility.

CHAPTER 13:
ETHICAL FOUNDATIONS OF AUTONOMOUS PRACTICE

Multiple Choice Answers

1. **B – Alignment of authority, responsibility, and accountability**

   Rationale: "The ethical foundation of autonomous practice rests on the alignment of authority, responsibility, and accountability." Not just regulation (A), not delegation (C), not experience (D). Ethical coherence requires alignment.

2. **B – Ethical misalignment and potential for unchecked harm**

   Rationale: "When authority is present but accountability is absent, the result is ethical misalignment with potential for unchecked harm." Authority without accountability is dangerous. Not autonomous practice (A), not delegation (C), not collaboration (D).

3. **B – Clinical competence and commitment to evidence-based standards**

   Rationale: "Beneficence within autonomous practice requires clinical competence, commitment to evidence-based standards, and sustained professional development." Not rigid protocols (A), not always deferring (C), not avoidance (D). Positive obligation to do good.

4. **B – Recognize limits and seek consultation when appropriate**

   Rationale: Nonmaleficence "extends to the responsibility to recognize the limits of one's expertise and to seek consultation or referral when patient needs exceed one's scope." Not avoiding complexity (A), not perfection (C), not defensive practice (D). Includes knowing limits.

5. **B – NPs provide evidence-based guidance respecting patient values and preferences**

   Rationale: Patient autonomy means "respecting patient values and preferences within the context of evidence-based recommendations and professional judgment." Not patients alone (A), not NP decides alone (C), not family over patient (D). Shared decision-making.

6. **B – Equitable access to competent autonomous care**

   Rationale: "Justice examines whether regulatory structures, scope limitations, or practice barriers create inequities in access to competent autonomous care." Not just legal compliance (A), not billing (C), not hierarchies (D). Fairness in access.

7. **B – Honest acknowledgment of limits, appropriate consultation, and ethical decision-making**

   Rationale: Professional integrity requires "honesty about limits, willingness to seek consultation, and commitment to ethical decision-making even when inconvenient." Not hiding uncertainty (A), not false confidence (C), not practicing beyond scope (D). Honesty and ethics.

8. **B – Inseparable, authority without accountability is ethically unsustainable**

   Rationale: "Authority and accountability are inseparable. Authority without accountability is ethically unsustainable." Central ethical principle. Not optional (A), beyond regulation (C), applies to all (D). Fundamental relationship.

9. **B – Competence, humility, and commitment to patient welfare over ego**

   Rationale: Ethical autonomous practice requires "competence, humility, and commitment to patient welfare above professional ego or economic interest." Not isolation (A), not just degrees (C), not just settings (D). Character and values matter.

10. **B – Consultation, referral, or acknowledgment of limitations**

Rationale: Ethics requires "consultation, referral, or transparent acknowledgment of limitations" when exceeding competence. Not proceeding anyway (A), not hiding (C), not pretending (D). Honesty and appropriate action.

Case-Based Application - Suggested Answers

Case Scenario 1:

Question 1: Authority-responsibility-accountability alignment: She has legal authority but limited experience creates gap between authority and competence. She's responsible for patient outcomes but may lack judgment to fully exercise accountability. Authority exists legally but ethical accountability requires competence to use it wisely. Legal ≠ ethical readiness.

Question 2: Ethical obligations despite legal authority: (a) Seek appropriate mentorship/preceptorship during transition, (b) Practice within competence even if authority exceeds it, (c) Consult frequently while building independent judgment, (d) Be transparent about experience level, (e) Pursue continuing education aggressively, (f) Prioritize patient safety over ego or income. Legal authority doesn't eliminate ethical obligation to practice competently.

Question 3: Ethical transition approach: (a) Negotiate for structured mentorship initially, (b) Start with patients within clear competence, (c) Build complexity gradually with oversight, (d) Establish collaborative relationships with experienced colleagues, (e) Maintain low threshold for consultation, (f) Document learning and competency development. Authority grows into with experience—legal permission isn't instant readiness.

Case Scenario 2:

Question 1: Tensions: (a) Beneficence (wanting to help) vs. nonmaleficence (avoiding harm from incompetence), (b) Patient autonomy (their choice of provider) vs. professional integrity (honest limits), (c) Justice (patient's access difficulties) vs. safety (appropriate expertise), (d) Compassion (understanding access barriers) vs. competence (recognizing boundaries). Multiple principles in conflict.

Question 2: Professional integrity requires: (a) Honest acknowledgment of limits to patient, (b) Not practicing beyond scope despite patient requests, (c) Explaining risks of managing unfamiliar condition, (d) Actively helping patient access appropriate specialist care, (e) Offering management within scope while coordinating specialist input. Integrity means honesty even when disappointing patient.

Question 3: Ethical approach: (a) Validate patient's access frustrations, (b) Honestly explain this exceeds training/expertise, (c) Help identify accessible specialist resources, (d) Offer to manage aspects within scope while deferring specialty-specific issues, (e) Provide care coordination, (f) Advocate for better access. Meeting patient needs ≠ practicing beyond competence. Can help without practicing outside scope.

True/False Answers

1. **FALSE** - "Authority without accountability is ethically unsustainable" regardless of legal permission. Ethics transcends regulation.
2. **TRUE** - "Professional integrity requires honesty about limits, willingness to seek consultation, and commitment to ethical decision-making."
3. **FALSE** - Beneficence means promoting patient welfare through evidence-based care, not just satisfying requests. May require difficult conversations.
4. **TRUE** - Justice "examines whether regulatory structures...create inequities in access to competent autonomous care."
5. **FALSE** - Ethics requires competence and consultation when needed, not perfection. Mistakes happen; ethical practice acknowledges and learns.

CHAPTER 14:
JUSTICE AND REGULATION

Multiple Choice Answers

1. **B – Fair equality of opportunity and benefit to the least advantaged**

   Rationale: Rawlsian justice emphasizes "fair equality of opportunity and arrangements that benefit the least advantaged members of society (the difference principle)." Not market forces (A), not revenue (C), not hierarchies (D). Justice for vulnerable.

2. **B – What regulatory system one would choose without knowing their position within it**

   Rationale: "The 'veil of ignorance' asks: what regulatory system would one design without knowing whether they would be a patient, NP, physician, or regulator?" Removes self-interest from policy design. Not training memory (A), not patient understanding (C), not credential hiding (D). Thought experiment about fairness.

3. **B – Benefit the least advantaged or improve overall access to care**

   Rationale: "The difference principle suggests that inequalities (such as scope restrictions) are justified only if they benefit the least advantaged." Restrictions must help vulnerable populations. Not physician income (A), not reducing NPs (C), not tradition (D). Must benefit those with worst access.

4. **B – Justice concern, barriers serving professional protection rather than public welfare**

   Rationale: When restrictions "fail to demonstrably improve patient outcomes or access" they raise "justice concerns, suggesting that barriers may serve professional protection rather than public welfare." Not caution (A), not evidence-based (C), not standard (D). Protectionism concern.

5. **B – Actually serve their stated purpose (patient safety) or primarily benefit incumbent professionals**

   Rationale: Justice analysis asks "whether restrictive scope regulations serve their stated purpose (patient protection) or function primarily to benefit incumbent professionals." Distinguishes public welfare from protectionism. Not physician employment (A), not complexity (C), not tradition (D). Purpose matters.

6. **B – Qualified professionals can practice to full scope without arbitrary barriers**

   Rationale: "Fair equality of opportunity suggests that qualified professionals should be able to practice to the full extent of their education and competence without arbitrary barriers that serve primarily to protect incumbent practitioners." Not everyone same (A), not market (C), not urban-focused (D). Removing unjustified barriers.

7. **B – Possible regulatory capture, protectionism rather than public welfare**

   Rationale: "When evidence demonstrates that autonomous NP practice is safe and effective, yet regulatory restrictions persist, this suggests regulatory capture, where policy serves incumbent professional interests rather than public welfare." Not evidence irrelevance (A), not caution (C), not uncertainty (D). Protectionism indicator.

8. **B – Do they improve access for underserved populations?**

   Rationale: Justice framework asks "do scope restrictions improve access for underserved populations, or do they worsen existing healthcare inequities?" Focus on vulnerable populations. Not market share (A), not bureaucracy (C), not tradition (D). Access for least advantaged.

9. **B – That autonomous practice can address healthcare access inequities**

   Rationale: Nursopathic medicine's justice argument is "that autonomous nurse practitioner practice, when aligned with competence and accountability, can address healthcare access inequities." Not superiority (A), not elimination (C), not just economics (D). Justice through access.

10. **B – Creates barriers that may worsen access for vulnerable populations**

    Rationale: Requiring collaboration "without evidence" it improves outcomes "creates barriers that disproportionately affect vulnerable populations in rural and underserved areas." Not prudent (A), not protective (C), not standard (D). Worsens inequity.

Case-Based Application - Suggested Answers

Case Scenario 1:

Question 1: Difference principle NOT met: Collaboration requirements harm the least advantaged (rural pregnant women). Restriction doesn't benefit them, worsens access, increases maternal mortality risk. Regulations benefit physicians (protecting market) but harm most vulnerable patients. Fails justice test. Restrictions should help worst-off, these harm them.

Question 2: Veil of ignorance: If designing policy without knowing whether you'd be: (a) Rural pregnant woman needing care, (b) Women's health NP wanting to practice, (c) Distant physician, (d) Regulator, what policy would you choose? Likely: allow competent NPs to practice where needed. Behind the veil, you'd prioritize access over professional protection since you might be the pregnant woman.

Question 3: Illustrates justice concerns: (a) Restrictions don't improve safety, they worsen access, (b) Harm falls on most vulnerable (rural, low-income, minority women often), (c) Policy serves incumbent physician interests (market protection) over public welfare, (d) Creates arbitrary barrier unrelated to competence, (e) Evidence shows WH NPs can provide safe prenatal care. Regulations creating worse outcomes for vulnerable = justice violation.

Case Scenario 2:

Question 1: Reveals: Restrictions don't improve quality (State B outcomes no better) but do worsen access (State B worse access). Physician arguments are "post-hoc justification" for protectionism—evidence doesn't support quality claims. Justice issue: vulnerable populations suffer from restrictions while physician interests are served. Policy divorced from evidence serves incumbents, not patients.

Question 2: Rawlsian analysis: (a) Restrictions don't benefit least advantaged, they harm them (worse access), (b) Don't improve outcomes. Fail to justify inequality, (c) Serve physician interests, regulatory capture, (d) Fail difference principle. Create inequality without benefiting vulnerable. When restrictions harm access without improving safety, they're unjust, serve professional protection, not patient welfare.

Question 3: Policymakers should ask: (a) What evidence supports these restrictions improving outcomes? (If none, why maintain them?), (b) How do restrictions affect access for underserved populations? (If worsening access, how is this justified?), (c) Who benefits from current policy—patients or incumbent professionals?, (d) What would regulatory structure look like if designed behind veil of ignorance?, (e) Are we serving public welfare or professional interests? Evidence-based justice analysis, not tradition or protectionism.

True/False Answers

1. **TRUE** - The "veil of ignorance" asks what system we'd choose "without knowing whether we would be a patient, NP, physician, or regulator."
2. **FALSE** - Claiming safety isn't sufficient, must actually improve outcomes. Without evidence, restrictions may serve protectionism, not safety.
3. **TRUE** - The difference principle says "inequalities (such as scope restrictions) are justified only if they benefit the least advantaged."
4. **TRUE** - Justice analysis "examines whether regulatory structures serve public welfare or function primarily to protect incumbent professional interests."
5. **FALSE** - Access is central to justice—"regulatory structures that limit access disproportionately affect vulnerable and underserved populations."

CHAPTER 15:
AUTONOMOUS PRACTICE AS NECESSITY

Multiple Choice Answers

1. **B – A structural and ethical necessity, not merely an aspirational goal**

   Rationale: The chapter argues that autonomous NP practice is a structural and ethical necessity — not aspirational, not geographic, and not contingent on workforce conditions. The ethical argument is that responsibility requires commensurate authority. The structural argument is supported by workforce data, access inequities, cost pressures, and decades of safety and effectiveness research.

2. **B – The principle that responsibility must be paired with commensurate authority**

   Rationale: The ethical case rests on the principle that responsibility must be paired with commensurate authority. An NP who is held accountable for clinical outcomes but lacks the authority to act on clinical judgment is placed in an ethically untenable position — responsible without being empowered. This misalignment is the ethical core of the chapter's argument.

3. **B – Continuity of care and patient safety**

   Rationale: Fragmented authority across the five domains primarily undermines continuity of care and patient safety. When a clinician who holds longitudinal knowledge of a patient — across acute episodes, chronic disease management, preventive care, and specialty needs — cannot act autonomously on that knowledge, the continuity that makes the five-domain model coherent is disrupted.

4. **B – Alignment of authority, responsibility, and accountability within collaborative systems**

   Rationale: Autonomy within nursopathic medicine is defined as the alignment of authority, responsibility, and accountability within collaborative systems — not as isolation from other professionals or freedom from oversight. The model explicitly assumes and values interdisciplinary collaboration. Autonomy of judgment coexists with, and operates within, those systems.

5. **B – Workforce data, access inequities, cost pressures, and decades of safety and effectiveness research**

   Rationale: The structural necessity argument is supported by converging evidence: workforce data documenting clinician shortages and NP availability, access inequities in underserved areas, cost pressures in healthcare systems, and decades of research demonstrating safe and effective autonomous NP practice. It is not based on anecdote, theory alone, or a single study.

6. **B – Coexist—autonomy of judgment operates within, not outside of, interdisciplinary systems**

   Rationale: Autonomous practice and collaboration coexist within nursopathic medicine. Autonomy of judgment — the capacity to make independent clinical decisions — operates within, not outside of, interdisciplinary systems. The NP consults, refers, co-manages, and coordinates with other professionals. None of that negates independent clinical accountability; it expresses it.

7. **B – Explaining how NPs practice medicine through an advanced nursing framework**

   Rationale: The book's primary theoretical contribution is explaining how NPs practice medicine through an advanced nursing framework — providing an internally coherent, nursing-centered account of what autonomous NP practice is and why it is coherent as nursing. It is not a scope advocacy document, a superiority argument, or a proposal for new licensure.

8. **B – Functional dimensions of autonomous practice that operate together in every clinical encounter**

   Rationale: The five domains represent functional dimensions of autonomous practice that operate together in every clinical encounter. They are not sequential career stages, distinct service lines, or hierarchical levels. An NP in any single encounter may be practicing across all five domains simultaneously — acute care, longitudinal management, preventive reasoning, interdisciplinary coordination, and specialty lens.

9. **B – When authority requires external approval before implementation, evidence-based interventions may be delayed or diluted**

   Rationale: The argument that autonomy is a condition for evidence-based practice means that when clinical authority requires external approval before implementation, evidence-based interventions may be delayed, modified, or foregone entirely. A clinician who cannot act on their clinical judgment without another professional's approval cannot fully implement best-evidence care when that approval is withheld or delayed.

10. **B – Nursing can and should explain its own advanced practice through internally coherent, nursing-centered frameworks**

    Rationale: The book's ultimate message is that nursing can and should explain its own advanced practice through internally coherent, nursing-centered frameworks. Rather than defending NP autonomy through equivalence arguments, historical precedent, or workforce necessity alone, the profession can articulate what autonomous NP practice is — from the inside — on nursing's own theoretical terms.

Case-Based Application - Suggested Responses

Case Scenario 1 – ICU/ED Staffing and Restrictive Regulations

How does this scenario illustrate both the structural and ethical necessity arguments?

Structural necessity: the workforce data is direct – ACNPs are present and qualified, physicians are unavailable, and patients will lose access to care if regulations are not revised. The structural argument does not require proving NPs are superior; it requires only that qualified clinicians are available and being prevented from practicing by regulatory requirements that serve no patient safety purpose in this context. Ethical necessity: ACNPs in this scenario are expected to be present and accountable for the clinical environment but lack the authority to act autonomously. They are responsible without being empowered – the exact ethical misalignment the chapter identifies. Requiring physician oversight that is physically unavailable does not enhance safety; it creates a fiction of oversight while eliminating actual care.

What are the access and safety implications?

Access: patients who would otherwise receive care from qualified ACNPs either receive no care or must be transferred, creating delay, cost, and risk. Safety: the alternative to autonomous ACNP practice in this scenario is not physician care – it is no care or reduced care. A restrictive regulation that prevents qualified clinicians from practicing in the absence of physician oversight does not protect patients when physician oversight is structurally unavailable; it abandons them.

How does the nursopathic framework explain why autonomous ACNP practice is the ethically coherent solution?

The ACNP is educated, certified, and prepared for precisely this clinical context – acute and critical care across the lifespan. Their authority derives from their nursing education and APRN certification, not from physician delegation. Nursopathic medicine explains that the ACNP practicing autonomously in this ICU or ED is exercising nursing authority – acute care nursing practice at the advanced level – not medicine borrowed from a physician who is not present. The ethical coherence lies in the alignment: the ACNP has the preparation, the accountability, and the clinical knowledge. The regulatory structure that withholds the authority is the anomaly, not the practice.

What does this case reveal about the relationship between regulatory design and patient outcomes?

It reveals that regulations designed without adequate consideration of structural healthcare realities can cause direct patient harm. A regulation that may have been designed to protect patients – by requiring physician oversight – produces the opposite effect when the physician is unavailable and the qualified NP is present. The nursopathic framework's argument is not that oversight is bad, but that regulatory structures should be evaluated by whether they actually serve patient safety in practice – which is a Rawlsian justice argument developed more fully in Chapter 14.

Case Scenario 2 – Experienced NP Questions the Value of the Framework

How would you explain the practical value of an explicit theoretical framework?

Individual clinical competence answers the question "can this NP take care of patients well?" A theoretical framework answers a different question: "what is this practice, why is it coherent as nursing, and how can it be explained, defended, and sustained at the professional level?" The NP practicing for 15 years has accumulated clinical skill – but when challenged in a legislative hearing, a credentialing committee, a scope of practice dispute, or a moment of professional identity doubt, clinical experience alone is not the answer. The framework provides the language, the theoretical structure, and the professional grounding that experience cannot.

What can a shared professional framework accomplish that experience alone cannot?

A shared framework provides collective professional language — a way for the entire NP profession to explain what it does from the inside, on nursing's own theoretical terms. Individual experience is personal and variable; a shared framework is portable and persistent. It allows NPs in different specialties, settings, and states to speak with a common theoretical voice about the nature of their practice. It provides a foundation for professional education, scope of practice advocacy, and research that is grounded in nursing theory rather than borrowed from medicine or justified only by pragmatic outcomes.

How does the nursopathic medicine model strengthen the profession beyond any single NP's practice?

The model provides a nursing-centered account of advanced practice that the profession can use to educate students, defend scope in regulatory environments, respond to critics, and develop research agendas. A single NP practicing competently for 15 years contributes to her patients. The nursopathic framework contributes to the profession as a whole — giving every NP, including those yet to be educated, a coherent account of what they are doing and why it is both nursing and medicine simultaneously, rather than an awkward hybrid of the two.

How does the framework address imposter syndrome, and why does that matter professionally and clinically?

Imposter syndrome in NP practice is not a personal failing — it is a predictable consequence of practicing with autonomous authority that the profession has not yet fully articulated. When a patient calls an NP "doctor," or when a legislative committee asks "is this nursing or medicine?," and the NP has no theoretical answer, the ambiguity gets internalized as doubt. The nursopathic framework resolves this: it explains what is happening in the clinical encounter, names it within nursing, and gives the NP the language to say "what you are seeing is nursopathic medicine" with clarity and without apology. A clinician who is confident in the theoretical basis of their practice is a more grounded, more effective, and more professionally resilient clinician. That confidence matters for patient care.

True/False Answers

1. FALSE

   Rationale: The chapter argues the opposite: autonomous NP practice is a structural and ethical necessity, not something optional or negotiable based on workforce conditions. The structural argument is supported by converging evidence, and the ethical argument rests on the principle that authority must align with responsibility — a relationship that does not become optional based on geography or circumstances.

2. TRUE

   Rationale: Necessity is grounded in both ethical coherence (authority must match the responsibility an NP already carries) and structural demands (workforce shortages, access inequities, safety data, and cost pressures). The two arguments reinforce each other: the structural case shows the need; the ethical case shows why meeting that need through autonomous NP practice is not just practical but morally required.

3. FALSE

   Rationale: The structural necessity of autonomous NP practice is not limited to rural areas. Urban underserved communities, safety-net hospitals, community health centers, and federally qualified health centers in all geographic settings face access challenges that autonomous NP practice addresses. The argument is based on the full body of workforce and access evidence, not a rural exception.

4. **TRUE**

   Rationale: Fragmentation of authority across the five domains disrupts the coherence of nursopathic practice. An NP who holds longitudinal knowledge of a patient across all five domains – acute episodes, chronic disease management, preventive care, interdisciplinary coordination, and specialty lens – but cannot act autonomously on that knowledge cannot deliver the integrated, patient-centered care the model describes. Fragmentation has real continuity and safety consequences.

5. **FALSE**

   Rationale: The evidence base does not support this claim. Research comparing autonomous NP practice to physician-led or supervised models in equivalent clinical contexts has generally found comparable patient outcomes, with NPs demonstrating high performance on quality and safety metrics. Restrictive practice regulations have not been shown to improve patient outcomes and in many contexts – particularly in underserved settings – are associated with reduced access to care.

REFERENCES

American Association of Colleges of Nursing. (2021). *The essentials: Core competencies for professional nursing education*. American Association of Colleges of Nursing.

American Association of Nurse Practitioners. (2024). *State practice environment*. https://www.aanp.org/advocacy/state

American Nurses Association. (2015). *Code of ethics for nurses with interpretive statements*. American Nurses Association.

APRN Joint Dialogue Group. (2008). *Consensus model for APRN regulation: Licensure, accreditation, certification and education*. National Council of State Boards of Nursing.

Beauchamp, T. L., & Childress, J. F. (2019). *Principles of biomedical ethics* (8th ed.). Oxford University Press.

Benner, P. (1984). *From novice to expert: Excellence and power in clinical nursing practice*. Addison-Wesley.

Bodenheimer, T., & Sinsky, C. (2014). From triple to quadruple aim: Care of the patient requires care of the provider. *Annals of Family Medicine, 12*(6), 573–576. https://doi.org/10.1370/afm.1713

Bryant-Lukosius, D., & DiCenso, A. (2004). A framework for the introduction and evaluation of advanced practice nursing roles. *Journal of Advanced Nursing, 48*(5), 530–540. https://doi.org/10.1111/j.1365-2648.2004.03235.x

Carper, B. A. (1978). Fundamental patterns of knowing in nursing. *Advances in Nursing Science, 1*(1), 13–23.

Clance, P. R., & Imes, S. A. (1978). The imposter phenomenon in high achieving women: Dynamics and therapeutic intervention.

Psychotherapy: Theory, Research & Practice, 15(3), 241–247. https://doi.org/10.1037/h0086006

Croskerry, P. (2002). Achieving quality in clinical decision making: Cognitive strategies and detection of bias. *Academic Emergency Medicine, 9*(11), 1184–1204. https://doi.org/10.1197/aemj.9.11.1184

Daniels, N. (2008). *Just health: Meeting health needs fairly*. Cambridge University Press.

Delaney, K. R., & Shattell, M. (2013). The state of psychiatric-mental health nursing: The Peplau legacy and current realities. *Journal of the American Psychiatric Nurses Association, 19*(5), 229–231. https://doi.org/10.1177/1078390313502549

Delamaire, M., & Lafortune, G. (2010). Nurses in advanced roles: A description and evaluation of experiences in 12 developed countries (OECD Health Working Papers No. 54). OECD Publishing.

DiCenso, A., Guyatt, G., & Ciliska, D. (2005). *Evidence-based nursing: A guide to clinical practice*. Elsevier Mosby.

Fairman, J. A., Rowe, J. W., Hassmiller, S., & Shalala, D. E. (2011). Broadening the scope of nursing practice. *New England Journal of Medicine, 364*(3), 193–196. https://doi.org/10.1056/NEJMp1012121

Grace, P. J. (2018). *Nursing ethics and professional responsibility in advanced practice* (3rd ed.). Jones & Bartlett Learning.

Hamric, A. B. (2012). Empirical research on moral distress: Issues, challenges, and opportunities. *HEC Forum, 24*(1), 39–49. https://doi.org/10.1007/s10730-012-9177-x

Hamric, A. B., Hanson, C. M., Tracy, M. F., & O'Grady, E. T. (2014). *Advanced practice nursing: An integrative approach* (5th ed.). Elsevier Saunders.

Institute of Medicine. (2011). *The future of nursing: Leading change, advancing health*. National Academies Press.

Interprofessional Education Collaborative. (2016). *Core competencies for interprofessional collaborative practice: 2016 update*. Interprofessional Education Collaborative.

Kahneman, D. (2011). *Thinking, fast and slow*. Farrar, Straus and Giroux.

Kleinpell, R. M., Scanlon, A., Hibbert, D., Ganz, F., East, L., Fraser, D., ... Beauchesne, M. (2014). Addressing issues impacting advanced nursing practice worldwide. *Online Journal of Issues in Nursing, 19*(2), Manuscript 5. https://doi.org/10.3912/OJIN.Vol19No02Man05

Kohn, L. T., Corrigan, J. M., & Donaldson, M. S. (Eds.). (2000). *To err is human: Building a safer health system*. National Academies Press.

Locke, J. (1980). *Second treatise of government*. Hackett Publishing. (Original work published 1689)

Meleis, A. I. (2018). *Theoretical nursing: Development and progress* (6th ed.). Wolters Kluwer.

Melnyk, B. M., & Fineout-Overholt, E. (2019). *Evidence-based practice in nursing & healthcare: A guide to best practice* (4th ed.). Wolters Kluwer.

National Council of State Boards of Nursing. (2008). *Consensus model for APRN regulation: Licensure, accreditation, certification & education*. National Council of State Boards of Nursing.

National Governors Association. (2012). *The role of nurse practitioners in meeting increasing demand for primary care*. National Governors Association.

National Organization of Nurse Practitioner Faculties. (2017). *Nurse practitioner core competencies content*. National Organization of Nurse Practitioner Faculties.

Naylor, M. D., & Kurtzman, E. T. (2010). The role of nurse practitioners in reinventing primary care. *Health Affairs, 29*(5), 893–899. https://doi.org/10.1377/hlthaff.2010.0440

Newhouse, R. P., Stanik-Hutt, J., White, K. M., Johantgen, M., Bass, E. B., Zangaro, G., ... Weiner, J. P. (2011). Advanced practice nurse outcomes 1990–2008: A systematic review. *Nursing Economics, 29*(5), 230–250.

Newton, I. (1675). *Letter to Robert Hooke* [Letter]. Royal Society Archives.

Peng, Y., Xiao, S.-W., Tu, H., Xiong, X.-Y., Ma, Z.-J., Xu, W.-J., & Cheng, T. (2022). The impostor phenomenon among nursing students and nurses: A scoping review. *Frontiers in Psychology, 13*, 809031. https://doi.org/10.3389/fpsyg.2022.809031

Peplau, H. E. (1952). *Interpersonal relations in nursing: A conceptual frame of reference for psychodynamic nursing*. G. P. Putnam's Sons.

Peplau, H. E. (1997). Peplau's theory of interpersonal relations. *Nursing Science Quarterly, 10*(4), 162–167. https://doi.org/10.1177/089431849701000407

Rawls, J. (1971). *A theory of justice*. Harvard University Press.

Rawls, J. (1993). *Political liberalism*. Columbia University Press.

Reeves, S., Pelone, F., Harrison, R., Goldman, J., & Zwarenstein, M. (2017). Interprofessional collaboration to improve professional practice and healthcare outcomes. *Cochrane Database of Systematic Reviews, 2017*(6), CD000072. https://doi.org/10.1002/14651858.CD000072.pub3

Sackett, D. L., Rosenberg, W. M., Gray, J. A., Haynes, R. B., & Richardson, W. S. (1996). Evidence based medicine: What it is and what it isn't. *BMJ, 312*(7023), 71–72. https://doi.org/10.1136/bmj.312.7023.71

Safriet, B. J. (2011). Federal options for maximizing the value of advanced practice nurses in providing quality, cost-effective health care. In Institute of Medicine (Ed.), *The future of nursing: Leading change, advancing health*. National Academies Press.

Tanner, C. A. (2006). Thinking like a nurse: A research-based model of clinical judgment in nursing. *Journal of Nursing Education, 45*(6), 204–211. https://doi.org/10.3928/01484834-20060601-04

Weed, L. L. (1968). Medical records that guide and teach. *New England Journal of Medicine, 278*(11), 593–600. https://doi.org/10.1056/NEJM196803142781105

World Health Organization. (2010). *Framework for action on interprofessional education and collaborative practice*. World Health Organization.

Note to Readers: This reference list represents foundational and contemporary scholarship relevant to the theoretical framework of nursopathic medicine. Readers should consult the most current editions and emerging literature as advanced practice nursing continues to evolve. Additional references specific to individual specialty practice areas, educational methodologies, and emerging evidence should be consulted as appropriate to areas of clinical focus and professional interest.

GLOSSARY OF KEY TERMS

Accountability: The obligation to accept responsibility for one's clinical decisions and their outcomes; a foundational principle requiring alignment with authority in autonomous practice.

Acute Care: A domain of nursopathic medicine encompassing rapid assessment, diagnostic reasoning, and timely intervention in response to emergent or time-sensitive conditions.

Acute Reasoning: The domain-specific cognitive process within Acute Care characterized by rapid assessment, pattern recognition, and time-sensitive decision-making; guided by the core clinical question: What is happening right now, and what must I do?

Anticipatory Reasoning: The domain-specific cognitive process within Preventative Care focused on identifying and mitigating risks before they manifest as acute or irreversible conditions; guided by the core clinical question: What harm can I foresee and prevent before it happens?

Autonomous Practice: Clinical practice characterized by independent decision-making authority, direct accountability for outcomes, and professional judgment exercised within regulatory scope without requiring external permission or supervision.

Chronic Care: A domain of nursopathic medicine characterized by sustained responsibility for monitoring, adjusting, and managing patient conditions over time with emphasis on continuity and longitudinal outcomes.

Clinical Reasoning: The cognitive processes through which nurse practitioners integrate biomedical knowledge, nursing judgment, patient context, and evidence to guide assessment, diagnosis, treatment, and management decisions.

Collaboration: Purposeful engagement with other healthcare professionals to enhance patient care through integration of expertise while maintaining clear professional boundaries and autonomous authority.

Conceptual Gap: The disconnect between the regulatory recognition of nurse practitioner autonomous practice and the theoretical explanation of how that practice functions within nursing; the central problem this book addresses.

Diagnostic-Therapeutic Practice Model: The practice model around which nursopathic medicine is organized, in which the clinician independently diagnoses, prescribes, treats, and longitudinally manages patients across the full cycle of care; the defining structure of nurse practitioner practice.

Evidence-Based Practice: The foundation of nursopathic medicine; clinical decision-making informed by current research, professional guidelines, and scientific evidence while remaining individualized to patient context.

Five-Domain Model: The organizational structure of nursopathic medicine consisting of five functional domains—Acute Care, Chronic Care, Preventative Care, Interdisciplinary Care, and Specialty Care—describing how nurse practitioners think and practice rather than where they work.

Hildegard Peplau (1909-1999): Psychiatric nurse theorist who developed the Interpersonal Relations theory, demonstrating that nurses could practice psychotherapy autonomously within a nursing framework. Her work established theoretical precedent for advanced practice nursing by showing how nursing could integrate activities from other disciplines (psychotherapy) while maintaining nursing identity through focus on therapeutic relationships and patient-centered care. Often called the "mother of psychiatric nursing."

Interdisciplinary Care: A domain of nursopathic medicine describing how nurse practitioners engage with multiple healthcare disciplines to optimize outcomes while preserving independent clinical authority and accountability.

Longitudinal Management: Clinical oversight and decision-making sustained across time and encounters; a defining feature of the Chronic Care domain.

Nursopathic Medicine: A conceptual framework explaining how nurse practitioners practice medicine autonomously through advanced nursing practice, organized around five functional domains supported by evidence-based practice. This framework applies specifically to nurse practitioner practice at the advanced practice registered nurse level and does not describe registered nursing practice, which operates under a different scope of practice, authority structure, and model of accountability.

Preventative Care: A domain of nursopathic medicine focused on risk identification, health optimization, and proactive intervention to prevent deterioration and promote functional outcomes.

Professional Formation: The structured development of clinical reasoning, ethical responsibility, and accountability required for autonomous practice through education and clinical experience.

Risk Stratification: The process of assessing and categorizing patient risk levels to guide the intensity and timing of preventive or therapeutic interventions.

Scope of Practice: The legally and professionally defined boundaries within which nurse practitioners may exercise clinical authority, established through licensure, certification, population focus, and practice context. Scope is determined by graduate education and national certification, not by employment setting. Autonomous practice must remain within one's certified scope, with consultation or referral when patient needs exceed one's area of competency. Employment in a specialty clinical setting does not expand a nurse practitioner's scope beyond their certification.

Specialty Care: A domain of nursopathic medicine in which population-focused or condition-focused expertise refines autonomous practice without fragmenting professional identity.

Specialty Lens Reasoning: The domain-specific cognitive process within Specialty Care in which population-focused or condition-focused expertise refines clinical assessment, diagnosis, and management without fragmenting professional identity; activates immediately upon patient contact and shapes reasoning across all other domains; guided by the core clinical question: How does my specialty context reframe everything I observe?

Therapeutic Relationship: The sustained professional relationship between nurse practitioner and patient that serves as both a source of clinical insight and foundation for shared decision-making, particularly in longitudinal care.

ADDITIONAL TERMS

Advanced Practice Registered Nurse (APRN): A nurse who has completed graduate-level education (master's or doctoral degree), obtained advanced clinical training, and holds national certification in a specialized area of nursing practice. APRNs include nurse practitioners, clinical nurse specialists, nurse anesthetists, and nurse midwives.

ASCVD: Atherosclerotic Cardiovascular Disease. A category of conditions involving the buildup of plaque in arterial walls, leading to coronary artery disease, stroke, and peripheral artery disease. ASCVD risk assessment guides preventative interventions in primary care.

Authority: The legitimate power to make clinical decisions, prescribe treatments, and manage patient care independently. In autonomous practice, authority must be aligned with responsibility and accountability to ensure ethical practice.

Basic Structure: A concept from Rawlsian justice theory referring to the fundamental institutions and systems that shape society, including laws, government, and major social institutions. Applied to healthcare, regulatory frameworks are part of the basic structure because they determine who can practice and under what conditions, affecting access and opportunity for all.

Beneficence: The ethical principle of acting in the patient's best interest and promoting their welfare. In autonomous NP practice, beneficence requires clinical competence, commitment to evidence-based standards, and ongoing professional development.

Biomedical Knowledge: The scientific understanding of human physiology, pathophysiology, pharmacology, and disease processes that nurse practitioners integrate with nursing judgment to guide autonomous diagnostic and therapeutic decision-making.

C-peptide: A laboratory test measuring endogenous insulin production by the pancreas. C-peptide levels help distinguish between Type 1 and Type 2 diabetes and can identify conditions like Latent Autoimmune Diabetes in Adults (LADA).

Certification: Official recognition by a national certifying body (such as ANCC or AANPCB) that a nurse practitioner has met predetermined standards of knowledge and competency in a specific population focus or specialty area. Certification is required for licensure and defines scope of practice.

Clinical Competence: The demonstrated ability to apply clinical knowledge, technical skill, and professional judgment effectively and safely across the range of clinical situations within one's scope of practice; maintained through ongoing education, practice, and reflective development.

Clinical Judgment: The interpretation and application of clinical data in the context of patient-specific circumstances, professional knowledge, and ethical responsibility; distinct from clinical reasoning in that judgment reflects the evaluative conclusions drawn from the reasoning process.

Co-management: A model of interdisciplinary care in which a nurse practitioner and another provider share ongoing clinical responsibility for a patient's condition, with each contributing distinct expertise while maintaining clear accountability for their respective clinical decisions.

Collaboration Agreement: A legal document required in some states defining the relationship between a nurse practitioner and a physician. The framework presented in this book distinguishes between clinical collaboration (professional consultation based on patient need) and regulatory collaboration (mandated oversight requirements).

Collaborative Practice: A model of healthcare delivery in which nurse practitioners and other professionals work together based on clinical need and mutual expertise, distinct from mandated collaboration agreements; characterized by voluntary professional engagement rather than regulatory requirement.

Competency: The demonstrated ability to safely and effectively perform clinical skills and apply clinical judgment within one's scope of practice. Competency requires ongoing maintenance through continuing education and practice.

Conceptual Framework: A theoretical structure that organizes and explains relationships among concepts. Nursopathic medicine serves as a conceptual framework for understanding autonomous NP practice through its five domains.

Consultation: The act of seeking expert opinion or specialized knowledge from another healthcare professional based on clinical need, not regulatory requirement. Consultation enhances autonomous practice and represents professional maturity, not limitation of authority.

Continuity of Care: The deliberate maintenance of coherent, coordinated care across time, settings, and providers. In the Chronic Care domain, continuity is an active process requiring intentional communication and clinical oversight, not a passive outcome.

Diagnostic Reasoning: The cognitive process of formulating working diagnoses based on clinical assessment, recognizing that diagnosis evolves as information accumulates over time rather than representing a discrete endpoint.

The Difference Principle: A concept from Rawlsian justice theory stating that social and economic inequalities are justified only if they benefit the least advantaged members of society. Applied to NP regulation, restrictive practice regulations must demonstrably improve access or outcomes for underserved populations to be ethically justified.

Differential Diagnosis: The systematic process of distinguishing among conditions with similar clinical presentations to arrive at the most likely diagnosis. This process requires thorough assessment, pattern recognition, and integration of multiple data sources.

Direct Primary Care (DPC): A healthcare delivery model in which patients pay a monthly membership fee directly to their primary care provider in exchange for comprehensive primary care services, without insurance billing. DPC emphasizes patient-centered care and relationship continuity.

Doctor of Nursing Practice (DNP): The terminal practice doctorate in nursing, preparing nurses for the highest level of clinical practice, leadership, and evidence-based practice implementation. Many NP programs now require or offer the DNP as the entry-level degree for advanced practice.

Epistemology: The branch of philosophy concerned with the nature, sources, and limits of knowledge. In nursing, epistemology addresses how clinical knowledge is constructed and validated, including the integration of empirical, aesthetic, personal, and ethical ways of knowing.

Fair Equality of Opportunity: A principle from Rawlsian justice theory requiring that positions and opportunities be genuinely open to all who are qualified. Applied to NP practice, this means that if nurse practitioners meet educational, certification, and competency standards, regulatory barriers not grounded in evidence of patient harm violate fair equality of opportunity.

Family Nurse Practitioner (FNP): A nurse practitioner certified in the family/individual across the lifespan population focus, prepared to provide comprehensive primary care to patients of all ages from birth through the end of life.

Five Domains: The functional dimensions of autonomous NP practice in nursopathic medicine: Acute Care, Chronic Care, Preventative Care, Interdisciplinary Care, and Specialty Care. These domains describe how NPs think and practice, not where they work.

Full Practice Authority: Regulatory status in which nurse practitioners can evaluate patients, diagnose conditions, order and interpret diagnostic tests, initiate and manage treatments, and prescribe medications without physician supervision or collaboration agreements. Also called "independent practice" or "unrestricted practice."

Harm Mitigation: Proactive strategies to prevent treatment-related adverse effects and iatrogenic complications. Extends beyond avoiding errors to include anticipating and preventing foreseeable harms from therapeutic interventions.

HbA1c (Hemoglobin A1C): A laboratory test measuring average blood glucose levels over the previous 2–3 months. HbA1c is used to diagnose diabetes and prediabetes, and to monitor long-term glycemic control in patients with diabetes.

Iatrogenic: Relating to illness, injury, or adverse effects caused by medical examination, treatment, or therapeutic intervention. In nursopathic medicine, iatrogenic risk awareness is integral to harm mitigation and informs both acute and longitudinal clinical decision-making.

Imposter Syndrome: The persistent feeling that one's professional authority is not legitimate despite objective evidence of competence. In nurse practitioners, imposter syndrome often reflects not personal inadequacy but a structural problem: the absence of theoretical language explaining how autonomous diagnostic and therapeutic practice functions within nursing. This framework addresses imposter syndrome by providing nursing-centered language for what nurse practitioners already do.

Independent Judgment: The exercise of autonomous clinical decision-making based on professional knowledge, evidence, and patient context without requiring external authorization; a defining feature of nurse practitioner practice within nursopathic medicine.

Independent Practice: See Full Practice Authority.

Interdisciplinary Reasoning: The domain-specific cognitive process within Interdisciplinary Care that recognizes when consultation, referral, or collaborative input would enhance patient care, while maintaining clear professional boundaries and autonomous accountability; guided by the core clinical question: When does another discipline's expertise enhance this patient's care?

Justice: The ethical principle of fairness in the distribution of benefits and burdens. In healthcare regulation, justice requires examining whether scope restrictions actually serve their stated purpose of patient protection or primarily benefit incumbent professionals.

LADA (Latent Autoimmune Diabetes in Adults): Sometimes called Type 1.5 diabetes, LADA is a form of autoimmune diabetes that develops in adults and progresses more slowly than classic Type 1 diabetes. Diagnosis requires evidence of autoimmune antibodies and progressive beta-cell failure.

Lantus: Brand name for insulin glargine, a long-acting basal insulin used in diabetes management. Lantus provides steady insulin coverage over approximately 24 hours and is often used in Type 1 diabetes, LADA, and advanced Type 2 diabetes.

Liberty Principle: A concept from Rawlsian justice theory holding that each person has an equal right to the most extensive basic liberties compatible with similar liberties for all. Applied to healthcare regulation, practice restrictions must be evaluated against the liberty interests of both practitioners and patients.

Licensure: Legal authorization granted by state boards of nursing allowing nurse practitioners to practice within a defined scope. Licensure requirements typically include graduate education, national certification, and ongoing continuing education.

Longitudinal Accountability: The sustained responsibility for monitoring, evaluating, and adjusting a patient's care over time; extending beyond individual encounters to encompass the cumulative trajectory of clinical outcomes across the full arc of the therapeutic relationship.

Longitudinal Reasoning: The domain-specific cognitive process within Chronic Care that unfolds across repeated encounters, recognizing patterns, trends, and deviations that emerge only through sustained observation over time; guided by the core clinical question: How has this patient changed over time, and how do I adjust?

Medical Diagnosis: The identification of disease, injury, or other pathological conditions. In nursopathic medicine, NPs engage in medical diagnosis while practicing through a nursing framework that emphasizes integrated assessment, patient context, and therapeutic relationships.

Mentorship: A sustained professional relationship in which an experienced clinician provides guidance, perspective, and developmental support to a less experienced practitioner beyond the formal educational period; the second mechanism of professional formation following preceptorship.

MoCA (Montreal Cognitive Assessment): A validated screening tool for detecting mild cognitive impairment and early dementia. The MoCA assesses multiple cognitive domains including memory, attention, language, and executive function, with scores ranging from 0–30.

Moral Distress: The psychological experience of knowing the ethically appropriate action but being unable to carry it out due to institutional, regulatory, or systemic constraints; a recognized challenge in autonomous practice environments where scope restrictions conflict with clinical judgment.

Nonmaleficence: The ethical principle of "first, do no harm." Includes the responsibility to recognize limits of expertise and seek consultation when patient needs exceed one's scope of competency.

Nurse Practitioner (NP): An advanced practice registered nurse educated at the master's or doctoral level, nationally certified in a population focus, and licensed to provide comprehensive healthcare services including diagnosis, treatment, and management of acute and chronic conditions.

Nursing Epistemology: The study of how nursing knowledge is generated, organized, and applied in clinical practice; encompasses empirical, aesthetic, personal, and ethical ways of knowing as described by Carper (1978) and provides the philosophical grounding for nursing-centered clinical reasoning.

Original Position: A concept from Rawlsian justice theory describing the hypothetical situation in which people choose principles of justice behind the veil of ignorance, before knowing their place in society. Used to evaluate what practice authority rules rational people would accept as fair.

Patient Autonomy: The ethical right of patients to make informed decisions about their own healthcare, including the right to accept, refuse, or modify recommended treatments; supported in nursopathic medicine through shared decision-making within the therapeutic relationship.

Pattern Recognition: The cognitive ability to rapidly identify clinical presentations based on experience and knowledge, allowing efficient decision-making under time constraints. Particularly important in the Acute Care domain.

Population Focus: The specific patient population for which a nurse practitioner is educated and certified (e.g., family/individual across lifespan, adult-gerontology, pediatrics, neonatal, women's health, psychiatric-mental health). Population focus, not employment setting, defines scope of practice.

Preceptorship: A structured clinical teaching relationship in which an experienced practitioner directly supervises and guides a student or new graduate through clinical practice, providing real-time feedback and modeling autonomous clinical reasoning; the first mechanism of professional formation.

Prescriptive Authority: Legal authorization for nurse practitioners to prescribe medications, including controlled substances (in most states). The scope of prescriptive authority varies by state and is an essential component of autonomous practice.

Professional Dignity: The inherent worth of the nurse practitioner role as a legitimate and autonomous profession; sustained through theoretical clarity, ethical practice, and the refusal to accept characterizations of NP practice as derivative or subordinate.

Professional Identity: The internalized understanding of oneself as a member of the nursing profession, shaped by education, values, ethical commitments, and scope of practice. Nursopathic medicine provides a framework for maintaining nursing professional identity while exercising autonomous clinical authority.

Public Justification: A principle from Rawlsian justice theory requiring that just institutions be explainable and defensible to citizens in terms they can reasonably accept, rather than through power or tradition alone. Applied to NP regulation, restrictive practice rules must be publicly justifiable on grounds other than incumbent professional interest.

Rawlsian Justice: Justice theory developed by philosopher John Rawls emphasizing fair equality of opportunity and arrangements that benefit the least advantaged. Applied in this book to evaluate whether NP practice restrictions serve public welfare or incumbent professional interests.

Referral: The transfer of clinical responsibility for a patient (or specific aspect of care) to another healthcare provider when patient needs exceed one's scope, expertise, or available resources. Appropriate referral demonstrates professional responsibility, not inadequacy.

Reflective Equilibrium: A concept from Rawlsian justice theory describing the process of adjusting principles and judgments to achieve coherence between general rules and specific cases. Applied to NP practice, it suggests that regulatory frameworks should evolve as evidence accumulates about the safety and effectiveness of autonomous practice.

Regulatory Capture: A situation in which regulatory policy serves the interests of incumbent professionals rather than public welfare. Occurs when restrictions on practice persist despite evidence they do not improve outcomes or access.

Restricted Practice: Regulatory status requiring nurse practitioners to practice under physician supervision or delegation, with significant limitations on autonomous authority. The most restrictive regulatory environment for NP practice.

RN-to-NP Transition: The developmental process through which a registered nurse acquires the knowledge, clinical reasoning capacity, and professional identity required for autonomous practice as a nurse practitioner; encompasses both formal graduate education and clinical formation through preceptorship.

Role Clarity: The clear articulation and mutual understanding of professional boundaries, responsibilities, and authority within and between healthcare disciplines; essential for effective interdisciplinary collaboration and for sustaining professional identity in shared clinical space.

Scope Alignment: The principle that a nurse practitioner's clinical activities must remain congruent with their certified population focus, graduate education, and demonstrated competency; with consultation or referral required when patient needs exceed scope boundaries.

Scope Creep: Pejorative term sometimes used to describe the expansion of NP practice authority. The framework in this book argues that autonomous NP practice represents appropriate use of graduate-prepared professionals' education and competency, not encroachment on medicine.

Shared Clinical Space: The domain in which nurse practitioners and physicians exercise overlapping diagnostic and therapeutic authority, creating conceptual tension about professional boundaries. Nursopathic medicine addresses this tension by explaining how NPs practice medicine through a nursing framework.

Shared Decision-Making: A collaborative process between the nurse practitioner and patient in which clinical evidence, professional judgment, and patient values and preferences are integrated to arrive at mutually agreed-upon care plans; a cornerstone of the therapeutic relationship in nursopathic medicine.

SOAP Note: Subjective, Objective, Assessment, Plan. A structured clinical documentation format used to organize patient encounter information; in nursopathic medicine, the SOAP note serves not merely as a charting convention but as a framework that reflects and reinforces domain-specific clinical reasoning.

Specialty Certification: National certification in a defined specialty area beyond basic NP certification (e.g., oncology nursing, cardiovascular nursing, diabetes education). Specialty certification documents advanced expertise in specific clinical domains.

Statutory Authority: Legal permission granted through state law (statutes) defining what nurse practitioners are authorized to do. Varies significantly by state and determines whether NPs have full, reduced, or restricted practice authority.

Supervision: Direct oversight of clinical practice by another healthcare provider, typically required in restricted practice states. Distinct from consultation, which is sought based on clinical need rather than regulatory mandate.

Therapeutic Reasoning: Clinical decision-making focused on selecting, initiating, monitoring, and adjusting treatment interventions while balancing standardization with individualization based on patient context and response.

The Veil of Ignorance: A thought experiment from Rawlsian justice theory asking what regulatory system one would design without knowing their position within it (patient, NP, physician, or regulator). Used in this book to evaluate the fairness of practice restrictions.

The Vine Metaphor: A visual metaphor from Chapter 11 representing interdisciplinary collaboration. When the vine is "too tight," excessive oversight constricts autonomous practice; when "too loose," care becomes fragmented. Balance requires thoughtful calibration of professional relationships.

ABOUT THE AUTHOR

Lazaro Gafas, MSN, APRN, FNP-C, PMHNP-BC, is a board-certified Psychiatric-Mental Health Nurse Practitioner and the founder of Miami Mental Health in Miami, Florida. He works with individuals from all walks of life, helping them navigate anxiety, depression, bipolar disorder, ADHD, insomnia, and other mental health challenges with clarity and compassion.

Lazaro's journey in healthcare began in primary care, where he learned the importance of seeing the whole person—not just a diagnosis. That foundation continues to shape his work today. He believes meaningful mental health care happens when people feel heard, respected, and supported with practical, evidence-based tools they can use in everyday life.

Through his practice and his writing, Lazaro is passionate about breaking the stigma around mental health and making psychiatric care more approachable and human. His work in developing the nursopathic medicine framework reflects his commitment to clarifying how nurse practitioners practice autonomously while maintaining the patient-centered values at the heart of nursing.

This book is dedicated to the memory of his mother, Osmara Borrero, whose struggle with mental illness and loss to suicide in 2019 profoundly shaped his understanding of the critical importance of accessible, expert psychiatric care. Her memory continues to inspire his advocacy for autonomous advanced practice nursing, particularly in mental health settings where timely, expert intervention can save lives.

Lazaro's goal is simple: to help people feel better, think more clearly, and move forward with confidence and hope—and to ensure that the nurse practitioners who provide that care have the professional frameworks, autonomous authority, and recognition they deserve.

INDEX

www.ingramcontent.com/pod-product-compliance
Lightning Source LLC
LaVergne TN
LVHW052112210926
848482LV00025B/551
* 9 7 9 8 9 9 4 7 6 0 1 0 9 *